Courage

COURAGE

*The Story of the Mighty Effort
to End the Devastating Effects
of Multiple Sclerosis*

by Richard Trubo

INTRODUCTION BY SYLVIA LAWRY
AFTERWORD BY MIKE DUGAN

Ivan R. Dee
CHICAGO 2001

Library of Congress Cataloging-in-Publication Data:
Trubo, Richard.
    Courage : the story of the mighty effort to end the devastating effects of multiple sclerosis / by Richard Trubo ; introduction by Sylvia Lawry ; afterword by Mike Dugan.
        p. cm.
    Includes index.
    ISBN 1-56663-414-8 (alk. paper)
        1. National Multiple Sclerosis Society (U.S.)—History.   2. Multiple sclerosis—United States.   I. Title.
    RA645.M82 T78 2001
    616.8'34'00973—dc21   2001037219

Contents

Acknowledgments

THIS BOOK charts the history of a movement that began more than five decades ago, launched and guided initially by one woman, Sylvia Lawry, whose lifetime mission became ending the suffering of people stricken with multiple sclerosis. In writing the history of an organization more than fifty years old, I relied on her and many other people who helped move this story from idea to printed page. They include:

Jane Dystel, my literary agent, who has extraordinary integrity, intelligence, and publishing savvy. She brought this book project to me, and I relied on her sage advice many times. I feel very fortunate to have worked with her for more than a decade.

Oscar Dystel, whose thoughtful suggestions in the project's final stages helped shape the manuscript into its final form.

General Mike Dugan, who was not only generous with his own insights into the contemporary MS movement but also made his dedicated staff at the National Multiple Sclerosis Society accessible for interviews and research assistance.

Martha King, who understood the complexity of this undertaking and was extremely helpful. Particularly in the early stages of this project, she graciously answered one question after another and introduced me to many people who would help me tell the story of the National MS Society.

Ben Sloane, who was enthusiastic about this book from the beginning. He orchestrated many small details related to this project and came to the rescue on numerous occasions.

The many people—physicians, families, and National MS Society staff—some of whose names appear throughout this book, who provided valuable information and insights. I am particularly indebted to people with MS who, directly or indirectly, taught me so much. From many parts of the country and from many walks of life, these courageous men and women shared their triumphs and struggles, and were wonderful teachers. Their strength and courage are inspiring, and they helped sculpt this story.

Sylvia Lawry, who cared enormously about people and their well-being, and whose commitment to defeating MS was a magnificent obsession. She persevered fearlessly for more than half a century and showed what determination can accomplish even in the face of a cruel, stubborn adversary. The personal sacrifices she made for every person with MS are documented throughout this book. In the midst of her unwavering war against the disease, she spent many long days with me, recollecting the role that she and the Society played in the effort to conquer MS. As this book moved from gestation to completion, she provided encouragement every step of the way and trusted me to tell the story as I saw it.

As the psychologist and philosopher William James wrote, "I will act as if what I do makes a difference." Sylvia Lawry made a difference.

RICHARD TRUBO

Foreword

THIS BOOK is the personal history of Sylvia Lawry, a tenacious, iron-willed crusader against one of life's most mysterious diseases, multiple sclerosis. First identified in the early nineteenth century, MS remained untreatable for more than 150 years— and even today its treatment is uneven and only episodically successful. But what has changed over the past 50 years is the extent to which people with MS, their families, the medical profession, and the scientific research community have been able to come to grips with the reality of MS. Treatment of MS is improving; knowledge of MS is proliferating; research funding is available to every MS researcher with a good idea; and the general public has become aware of MS as a devastating disease but one with which those who are afflicted can cope successfully.

If there is one individual who can claim credit for this progress, and the creation and training of thousands upon thousands of highly motivated volunteers, that individual is Sylvia Lawry. As a young woman whose brother, Bernard, was an MS victim, she built the National Multiple Sclerosis Society (the NMSS) brick by brick through dedication and pure grit. It was primarily her vision that resulted in the establishment of the National Institute for Neurological Diseases and Blindness, one of the important government funders, within the National Institutes of Health, of basic research in neurological diseases. No corporate chieftain was safe from her assault. No medical researcher or practitioner could turn aside her plea for help. And woe to the volunteer in the trenches once Sylvia fixed her sights on what that volunteer could do in the fight against MS.

Successful corporate leaders such as Dan Haughton of Lockheed and John McGillicuddy of Manufacturers Hanover; show business showstoppers such as Shirley Temple Black and Frank Sinatra; leading physicians such as Dr. Houston Merritt and Dr. Tracy Putnam; and Sylvia's successors as NMSS CEOs, Thor Hanson and Mike Dugan, all bent to her will and followed her lead in helping to raise money, conduct research, motivate volunteers, and increase awareness.

In her later years, after turning leadership of the NMSS over to Thor Hanson in the 1980s and until her death early in 2001, Sylvia energized the International Federation of Multiple Sclerosis Societies (the IFMSS), recruiting such worthy leaders as James Wolfensohn and James Cantalupo, and successfully persuading NMSS board members such as William Benton and George Boddiger to expand their interests and their energies to help the IFMSS.

Although primarily Sylvia's biography, this book is also a chronicle of the National Multiple Sclerosis Society as seen through Sylvia's eyes. Filled with personal reminiscences and anecdotes, it is replete with instances of how Sylvia was able to overcome this and that challenge in advancing the fortunes of the Society. The book's description of the early years of the Society is especially fascinating as it describes the painstaking and sure-handed persistence of a young woman, without influence or resources, as she almost single-handedly gave birth to a national health agency.

For those of us who have spent important time in the fight against multiple sclerosis over the past fifty years, this book brings back fond memories. For anyone thinking about founding a national health agency to fight an unknown disease, to engage the medical research community in that fight, to motivate thousands of volunteers to become foot soldiers in that fight, and to raise increasing amounts for patient care and research now approaching $200 million per year, this book must be read.

PALMER BROWN
President and Chairman, NMSS, 1973–1978

CLIFFORD H. GOLDSMITH
Chairman, NMSS, 1984–1987

GEORGE J. GILLESPIE, III
Chairman, NMSS, 1987–1991

Introduction

BY SYLVIA LAWRY

". . . to take arms against a sea of troubles
and by opposing end them."
—*Hamlet*

THOSE FIGHTING WORDS from William Shakespeare have
been a source of inspiration for me since the earliest days of
the National MS Society. I still find this quote very meaningful,
keeping me focused on battling the devastating disease of multiple sclerosis alongside many thousands of volunteers who
have expended so much energy and fought so hard for so long.
Before the Society took on its current name many years ago, I
called it the Association for the Advancement of Research on
Multiple Sclerosis—or the acronym AARMS—again a reference
to the call to arms in *Hamlet*. What motivated me in the beginning, and still does today, is a powerful desire to see multiple
sclerosis eradicated. To my great disappointment, we haven't
yet found a cure and wiped out this invasive disease once and
for all. But we continue to fight the good fight—and I'm con-
fident that we will be victorious.

At times over the years, when people from all walks of life urged me to write a book about the battle against multiple sclerosis, I always rejected the idea, feeling it wouldn't be appropriate to tell the story of the National MS Society and the worldwide MS movement until we had achieved our final objective. But the book now in your hands serves a valuable purpose in that I believe it can help the public understand what has transpired in pursuit of our goal, and how we are coming closer to the final answer with each passing day. Also, it provides a window into the inner workings of the MS movement and counteracts a public misconception, voiced by many, that health agencies are self-serving and seek only to perpetuate themselves. Instead this book conveys a strong sense of commitment, integrity, and singleness of purpose.

Most recently, medications have become available that can alter the course of multiple sclerosis for the first time, providing dramatic benefits for hundreds of thousands of people with the disease. Even though there is more to be accomplished, I am comforted that the lives of so many men and women are better today than they would have been were it not for the National Society, the researchers, and the many volunteers who form our organization's backbone.

Those volunteers have meant so much to this movement. The media are filled with stories each day of man's inhumanity to man. This book, however, is a story of man's humanity to man. So much occurs in our world that demonstrates the compassion and caring of men, women, and children everywhere, yet these acts of kindness often go unrecognized and unappreciated. This book provides an inside look at an organization in which the positive actions of men, women, and children directly influence the quality of life of others. The volunteers of the National MS Society have shown, day after day, year after year, the good that can come when people are committed to making a difference. They have demonstrated what volunteers can accomplish when they have no personal agenda other than to improve the well-being of others, simply out of the goodness of their hearts.

Throughout the years I have frequently thought about the observations of Alexis de Tocqueville, the French statesman who visited the United States about two centuries ago and observed that Americans are "strange people." According to de Tocqueville, when these "strange" Americans are confronted with a common problem, they band together and form an association to deal with it. The National MS Society is a perfect example of what de Tocqueville wrote about—people banding together to conquer a vicious disease and improve the lives of people afflicted with it. As we've learned, these characteristics aren't unique to Americans. As the number of MS societies has grown throughout the world, people everywhere have reacted the same way when faced with this common problem. Persons with MS, their families, and communities at large have recognized that there is strength in numbers, and they have come together to fight this stubborn but beatable enemy.

I have often thought of the MS movement as a human laboratory in which people from every corner of the globe are working together in a shared mission. So many individuals from so many cultures have found that despite the differences in their backgrounds and the varying courses that their lives have taken, they can work together in harmony. The National MS Society and the International Federation of Multiple Sclerosis Societies have been recognized as model voluntary health agencies. This book tells the story of why these organizations are viewed with such admiration throughout the world.

What has kept me fighting for so long? My mentor during

the establishment of the National MS Society was Basil O'Connor, the head of the National Foundation for Infantile Paralysis that was so instrumental in the development of the polio vaccine. He and his staff explained to me that one day everything at the Foundation was business as usual, then the next day the electrifying news arrived that the Salk vaccine had provided deliverance from the scourge of polio. That same turn of events could occur with multiple sclerosis at any time as a result of the army of dedicated scientists and physicians worldwide who are focused on finding the answer to MS. Their hard work continues to give me hope that the ultimate answer to MS will come in the foreseeable future.

Much has been said about my own accomplishments and those of the National Multiple Sclerosis Society. None of these achievements would have been possible without the unwavering support of people from virtually every segment of society—men, women, and children, persons with MS, their friends and family members, as well as many other individuals who have been touched deeply by the courage of those who struggle with the disease every day. All of these people are the real heroes in the fight to defeat MS. Many of them have been recognized in the pages of this book; they have helped me and the movement in so many ways. But there are many others not mentioned who have made contributions that have been just as important and are just as deserving of my thanks.

I must recognize the medical and scientific volunteers for their invaluable contributions. Early on, the National MS Society flourished because its first Medical Advisory Board was composed of leaders in the neurological and public health specialties. This enabled us to recruit lay volunteers of comparable stature. Throughout the years, members of the Society's medical and scientific advisory boards (as well as members of comparable boards of other MS societies worldwide) have volunteered their time and expertise, serving on peer review and other scientific committees.

A tribute must also be bestowed upon the Society's professional and support staff, and the way in which they have supported our volunteer leadership. Many of those in this dedicated group became thoroughly committed to the cause and served in volunteer capacities in addition to their professional responsibilities. A great number of them remained as volunteers following their formal retirement. Some of these National MS Society staff members—past and present—have demonstrated an extraordinarily long-term commitment to the cause.

In the preparation of this book, I and many people in the MS movement participated in interviews conducted by Richard Trubo and others over several years. The author also spent countless hours researching names, events, and dates. I am grateful to all of those who took part in this interview and research process.

I wish to extend special recognition to Judith Price, a longtime colleague on the National MS Society staff, who had been in charge of many files and documents associated with the National Society and International Federation for more than twenty-five years. During the final preparations for this book, Ms. Price sorted through thousands of documents to find those most relevant to this project. She turned them over to Beverly Timberlake, another longtime National Society colleague, who typed many summaries that then were passed on to the author. I am grateful for these efforts by Ms. Timberlake.

Finally, I extend my special gratitude and appreciation to

the present volunteer and professional heads of the National Multiple Sclerosis Society and the International Federation of Multiple Sclerosis Societies:

Richard Slifka, chairman, National MS Society Board of Directors;

General Mike Dugan, U.S. Air Force, retired, president and CEO, National MS Society;

Dr. Stanley van den Noort, chairman, National MS Society Medical Advisory Board;

Peter Schweitzer, president, International Federation of MS Societies;

Christine Purdy, chief executive, International Federation of MS Societies;

Professor W. Ian McDonald, chairman, International Federation of MS Societies' International Medical Advisory Board.

Recognition is also due to many others, including volunteers and staff, who performed—and continue to perform—outstanding service on the local, national, and international levels. Space limitations prevent a listing of these names. The MS movement would not have accomplished all that it has if it did not have the support of these dedicated people.

Courage

Prologue

This book is a history of the multiple sclerosis movement, the organization and the people behind it. It is a medical detective story that has kept dedicated scientists working overtime in their laboratories searching for clues to unravel one of the more baffling and stubborn medical mysteries of our time. It is also the story of one woman and her brother, and the thousands of volunteers who have become the mettle of the National Multiple Sclerosis Society and the Multiple Sclerosis International Federation.

Until her death in February 2001, Sylvia Lawry was as committed to solving the puzzle of multiple sclerosis as she had been more than fifty years earlier. In her office at the Society's headquarters she was surrounded by photographs, plaques, and mementos that marked her many accomplishments. She worked tirelessly, focusing on the challenges of the moment while reflecting upon the achievements and disappointments of the past.

"When the Society was organized," she recalled, I was really walking into the unknown. There certainly was no assurance of success. I didn't know where my efforts would lead. But when I would get letters or phone calls from anguished people with MS, or from their family members, I was sustained by the knowledge that I had to try. I had to do something. The need that I felt to succeed was tremendous."

Amid pressures to meet the demands of its members over the years, the National MS Society has sometimes endured organizational growing pains, conflicts, and controversy. There have been heated internal debates over the respective roles of the local chapters and the national headquarters. There have been times when the financial stability of the organization has been threatened. There has been dissension over how funds should be appropriated. How much should be spent on services for people coping with MS? How much should be spent on research to find answers to the lingering mysteries of the disease?

Through it all, Sylvia Lawry was the glue that held the Society together. Her half-century commitment to the fight against MS helped downplay disappointments and smooth ruffled feathers while keeping the Society's goals on track.

She also took the MS movement to the world. This disease, she reasoned, knows no boundaries or borders. Few parts of the world are MS-free. More than 2.5 million people and their families are affected by multiple sclerosis the world over. Sylvia helped MS leaders in several countries found their own national societies. By the year 2000, the International Federation of Multiple Sclerosis Societies (recently renamed the Multiple Sclerosis International Federation) had grown to a 38-nation network with hundreds of thousands of volunteers. In MS Society chapters throughout the world, phones ring constantly. Some callers, anxious and anguished, have just been diagnosed with MS and are desperate for information. Others have had the disease for decades and are facing exacerbations or new loss of ability. After more than fifty years, the questions to the Society from the public are familiar, yet each one deserves individual attention. "Where can I go for the services I need?" "Is there anything that can be done for me?"

The information provided by the National MS Society fills a long-standing void. Alida Camp, a longtime MS Society Board member, had never heard of MS when her husband, Frederic, was diagnosed in the mid-1940s. Their doctor was reassuring but less than hopeful: "There's not very much we know about it, and there's not much we can do. But your husband shouldn't have too much trouble if he just takes it easy."

The Camps followed his advice, and Mr. Camp avoided strenuous activity. Shortly after receiving the diagnosis, however, his symptoms took a dramatic turn for the worse while the couple was vacationing in Williamsburg, Virginia. "As we finished our meal in the hotel restaurant," Alida said, "Fred stood up, and then he said, 'I can't walk.' He didn't seem to be kidding, and I immediately became very worried. But in a wifely fashion I said, 'Don't be silly, dear. Of course you can walk.' He looked at me with anxiety on his face, and he said, 'No, I'm sorry, I can't walk.' I had him lean on me, and we somehow made it out of the restaurant, and then I called for some help from the hotel manager. Two men helped Fred walk up the stairs to our room, and they put him in bed. I called our doctor right away, but he didn't seem overly concerned. He told me, 'Sometimes this happens. He'll be all right in a day or two.' Well, a few days went by, and he wasn't all right. We got him a wheelchair, and made the best of it." From that time forward, the Camps knew they were dealing with a very serious disease.

At the time when Frederic Camp learned of his disease, doctors often advised withholding the diagnosis from patients.

When Society Chairman Emeritus L. Palmer Brown was told that his wife had MS, their doctor said, "Your wife is a smart, educated woman, and she reads a lot. If we tell her she has MS, she's going to read up on it, and she'll find out that her problem can't be fixed and that the later stages of the disease can be very difficult. My suggestion is that you tell no one—not your wife or any other family member. Keep it to yourself."

Sylvia Lawry and those associated with the National MS Society have always felt an urgency growing out of the devastated lives that the disease leaves in its wake. MS Society psychologist Nicholas LaRocca notes, "MS affects more than the ability to walk. It can change the way people feel about themselves, the way they think, and their capacity to learn and remember."

These emotional and cognitive effects are not as visible as a wheelchair or a cane, but for many persons with MS they are the most pressing problems associated with the disease. Psychologists Paul J. Donoghue and Mary E. Siegel note that people with MS are often tormented with thoughts such as "I feel isolated from the rest of the world. . . . I feel like damaged goods. . . . How can I be competent feeling the way I do? . . . Who wants to employ someone who might be ill all of the time? . . . Did I cause this illness? . . . If I had eaten more or exercised more, would I be well today?"

Nancy Law, vice president for Client Programs for the National MS Society, told *Inside MS* in 1999, "MS can be a very lonely experience, especially at first. Few of your acquaintances have had the same experience. MS is tough on self-esteem and image, and sometimes you just don't know who you are anymore."

Though Sylvia Lawry's commitment to finding a solution to MS never faltered, she died without knowing the answers to key questions. The cause of MS remains unknown. There is no cure. Crucial strides have been made, many due to the efforts of the MS Society, and multiple sclerosis is much better known today than it was fifty years ago, but it remains a formidable foe.

The disease is no longer a secret, however. Well-known personalities such as actress Annette Funicello, TV host Montel Williams, and federal prosecutor Joseph Hartzler have openly acknowledged their disease while leading active and public lives. These high-profile individuals give courage to the thousands of ordinary people beset by the disease. It is this community that has formed the backbone of the MS Society. Thanks to the dedication of thousands of individuals, persons with MS and their families benefit every day from the services and programs of National MS Society chapters. They utilize information resources and local referrals. They are helped by professional counseling as well as by peer support, sharing their successes and their disappointments. They enjoy the improvements in equipment—from lightweight wheelchairs to accessible vans to electric door openers—that have made daily living easier. They reap the rewards of the Society's aggressive advocacy campaigns, including its relentless lobbying of Congress and state legislatures on their behalf. These same individuals contribute their energies and money to MS fundraisers, including golf tournaments, walks, fashion shows, bike tours, and concerts. They contact their legislators and solicit potential contributors. They distribute MS literature at health fairs and public gatherings. They are responsible for generating the dollars that buy microscopes and laboratory slides. When the MS Society was founded, there was almost no research into the disease. Today, apart from the U.S. government, the Society is the world's largest source of MS-related research funds. This money is channeled into cutting-edge studies in areas such as immunology and genetics. Many of the country's brightest scientists and physicians have become involved in MS research through Society-funded fellowships and research training programs.

Multiple sclerosis is a daunting adversary. Every hour of every day someone is told that he or she has the disease. MS patients in the United States alone total more than 300,000. As Sylvia Lawry often said, "Someone you know has MS." The disease strikes hard—physically, emotionally, and financially. A recent Society-sponsored study revealed that the average person with MS suffers costs approaching $44,000 per year. Of that, $21,500 goes to health-care expenses, and $21,700 is lost wages.

The story of the National Multiple Sclerosis Society and the international MS movement is still unfolding. The diagnosis of MS remains very disturbing, but people with MS can rightfully feel more empowered than ever before. Though mysteries surrounding MS remain unsolved, it is now a treatable disease. Recently approved drugs such as Betaseron, Avonex, and Capaxone specifically target the underlying disease, not just its symptoms. The drugs have successfully shattered the belief that nothing can be done about MS.

From the Society's modest beginnings, when Sylvia Lawry worked from sunrise to exhaustion in a donated eight-by-ten-foot office at the New York Academy of Medicine, the Society has grown dramatically. By 2000 it had expanded to a network of 140 local chapters and branches in every state. The ranks of members and volunteers increased to almost one million. Today the Society is the world's largest center for credible information about MS. What Sylvia Lawry created through her personal drive and boundless energy has been instrumental in helping many thousands of people with MS feel hope instead of hopelessness.

1

O N THE MORNING of May 1, 1945, a personal ad appeared
in the *New York Times*.

"Multiple Sclerosis. Will anyone recovered from it please
communicate with patient."

It was a small ad tucked into the Public Notices section of
the *Times* classifieds. But for the anguished young woman who
placed the ad, there was a real urgency to her plea. Her name
was Sylvia Lawry, and her brother, Bernard, had been diagnosed with multiple sclerosis. Together they were desperate for
answers to his disease.

Sylvia and her brother waited anxiously for replies.
Bernard was only twenty-one when he had been diagnosed with
MS several years before. His doctor had told him that MS was
very rare and that nothing could be done to treat it. As Bernard
began to struggle with the disease, he and Sylvia were disturbed
by how little modern medicine could offer him. They hoped
the notice in the *Times* might put them in touch with someone
who had found a way to produce a remission, a method that
Bernard could follow.

Within days of the ad's appearance, Sylvia began receiving responses—fifty-four in all—from MS sufferers or their family members. None spoke of a cure. Most were in the same predicament. They wanted information—any information—about this mysterious disease, and they asked her to send whatever she uncovered. All of them were anxious for help. All were desperate for some shred of hope.

Though the personal ad resulted in no concrete help for Bernard, it was the start of a new life for Sylvia. That summer, as the country rejoiced in the conclusion of World War II, she made plans for aggressive combat of her own. It was obvious to her that an association of some kind was necessary to bring MS sufferers together and somehow to draw the attention of the medical world to this disease. Bernard and the many other victims of MS needed more than the grim declaration that nothing could be done for them.

Sylvia Lawry had no medical background, no wealth, no social standing. She was a lonely but determined thirty-year-old woman who felt she had no choice but to help her brother. Bernard's condition, his motor skills and mobility, were worsening. It was agonizing for Sylvia to see him decline. A cure had to be found. Multiple sclerosis had to be recognized as a scourge that struck down young, vigorous people and robbed them of their futures.

Much of Sylvia's frustration was caused by how little was known about MS in 1945. Far from being rare, it was and is one of the most common diseases of the central nervous system. It is generally believed that people inherit a genetic susceptibility to MS and that it is triggered by any number of yet unknown environmental factors, possibly connected to viral agents. It is considered to be an autoimmune disorder. With MS, the immune system goes haywire, attacking the myelin sheathing that protects the nerve fibers of the brain and the spinal cord. Myelin is the protective coating of nerves, functioning not unlike the coating on telephone or electrical wires. If the coating wears thin, the wires are exposed and vulnerable to damage and short circuiting. When any part of the myelin sheathing is destroyed, nerve impulses to and from the brain may be distorted or interrupted. Some may never be transmitted at all. Such distortion of nerve impulses triggers MS symptoms. Some are so mild as to be unnoticeable. Other are so severe that the individual may be incapacitated. Though not considered terminal, MS can shorten lifespan if complications are poorly managed.

And the disease never disappears.

Little of that information was available to Sylvia when she began researching her brother's condition in the summer of 1945. She was frustrated by the scarcity of data, even in medical libraries. MS was all but unknown to the general public and a mystery to most physicians. Other chronic diseases such as cancer, heart disease, polio, and tuberculosis had much higher profiles, not to mention research and public awareness campaigns directed against them.

The first credible account of multiple sclerosis dates to 1822, when the English nobleman Sir Augustus Frederic d'Este, a cousin of Queen Victoria, wrote in his diary of a "curious malady" from which he suffered. His symptoms were familiar to MS sufferers: blurred vision, problems of balance, numbness, paralysis, weakness, and bladder trouble. D'Este traveled throughout Europe seeking relief from his illness which had no name, no known cause, and no treatment. He died at the age of fifty-four after a twenty-six year battle with the disease.

At the same time a number of doctors were beginning to take notice of what would ultimately be identified as MS. In

1839, the French physician Jean Cruveilhier detected spots or "brown patches" on the spinal cord of a woman during an autopsy. He described the spots as "islands of sclerosis," and he wrote that they were different than "any other morbid tissue of which I have knowledge." The name multiple sclerosis means, literally, many scars.

Nearly thirty years later, the French neurologist Jean Martin Charcot provided the first detailed description of multiple sclerosis. Charcot's housekeeper had experienced tremors, slurred speech, and vision difficulties, and although Charcot noted some parallels between her symptoms and those of Parkinson's disease, he believed he was observing a separate medical condition. He noted that this woman, and other patients, often had exacerbations or acute attacks of their symptoms followed by remissions when the symptoms subsided. He also observed that symptoms varied from one person to another. When autopsies were performed, scars or "plaques" were found throughout the central nervous system. Charcot gave the disease the name *sclerose en plaques,* and attempted to treat it with electrical stimulation and injections of gold and silver. He was perplexed by its resistance to everything he tried.

Since Charcot's time, researchers have debated whether multiple sclerosis was a new disease that emerged in the early 1800s or whether for centuries it had simply been overlooked or mislabeled. Its symptoms, however, are distinct: impaired movement and coordination, numbness and tingling, speech abnormalities, visual disorders, and impaired mental function. These symptoms range from mild to severe to incapacitating. The disease is two to three times more common in women, though it may be more severe in men. By 1945, when Sylvia and Bernard were desperately looking for answers to Bernard's condition, MS sufferers were regularly misdiagnosed. Patients went from doctor to doctor, often over a period of years, before the symptoms were correctly analyzed. Many were told that they were overworked and run-down and simply needed to make changes in their way of life. Others were advised that the illness was psychosomatic and that they should consult a psychiatrist. Still others were told they had brain tumors, pernicious anemia, encephalitis, or had suffered a stroke.

Even when the disease was properly diagnosed, doctors offered no treatment. Sylvia Lawry came to know well a sense of frustration, even futility among doctors when confronted with an MS patient. "Most neurologists weren't interested in seeing MS patients," she recalled. "They had little to offer beyond making the diagnosis. Many doctors were quite pessimistic. Their feeling was that nothing could be done for people with MS, and that they should just go home and wait to die."

Such attitudes made Sylvia all the more resolute to do something. As Bernard struggled with the disease, she became convinced that the research capabilities of modern medicine had to be applied to MS. Answers to its mysterious cause and its unpredictable path had to be found in laboratories. Scientists had to better understand the central nervous system and find out what factors made a particular individual susceptible to the disease. They had to research myelin and discover why it was selectively destroyed by the immune system and what triggered these attacks. They had to learn why the disease primarily struck young adults. They had to answer the riddle of why the disease ebbed and flowed, why it afforded remissions and struck with dreaded relapses.

Sylvia rued the fact that her brother Bernard, her friend and protector, had a disease that no one seemed to know anything about. She could not sit back and watch it destroy him. "His need is what stirred me," she said.

2

BORN TO IMMIGRANT PARENTS in Brooklyn in 1915, Sylvia was the oldest of four children. Her father, Jacob, had studied music in Europe, but at the turn of the century he set aside his dreams of becoming a classical violinist and went off to America. There he met and married Sophie, and went to work manufacturing bathing suits. "He was a workaholic before workaholic was even a word. He took his family and his role as a provider very seriously," Sylvia remembered.

Jacob Friedman was quiet and withdrawn, by no means a communicator, yet he surprised people with his knowledge of literature, classical music, and the arts. He avidly read the *New York Times, Collier's,* and the *Saturday Evening Post.* He stocked the family's bookshelves with the works of Shakespeare, Dickens, Washington Irving, and Bret Harte. A baby grand piano stood prominently in the family room, and the best music teachers were sought out to instruct the children.

Sophie was warm, spirited, and resourceful. She had a love of nature, but it paled next to her love for her family, which she once feared she might never have. After surgery to remove a tumor, she was told she might not be able to bear children. Four successful pregnancies—producing Sylvia, Bernard, Alice, and Lillian—dispelled that notion, and she threw herself whole-heartedly into motherhood. When invited to social events, she would attend only if the children could accompany her.

But in the years after the birth of her fourth child, Sophie developed clinical depression (her doctors labeled it "melan-cholia"), and she became unable to look after her family. As a result, Sylvia, at age fourteen, found herself in charge of the household. She had to prepare meals, do the laundry for the entire family, and raise sisters Alice and Lillian, then ages four and eight. "My life became geared to meeting responsibility. Because of my mother's illness, and with my father at work, I became the head of the household. I felt responsible for my mother, father, brother, and young sisters," Sylvia said.

Taking charge was nothing new to her. The family liked to tell the story of when they were living in the Bronx and Sylvia was only eight years old when she saw two men fighting in the street. A crowd of onlookers cheered them on. Sylvia, however, ran between them and shouted, "Stop it! Stop it! You're going to hurt yourselves." Stunned and perhaps embarrassed by the child's bold behavior, the two men lowered their fists and the fight was over.

As children, Sylvia and Bernard grew very close to each other. Bernard was shy but had a sweet personality that at-tracted people to him. After school and on weekends he helped out in the family's manufacturing business. Like his fa-ther, Bernard was drawn to books and developed a hunger for reading. As a teenager he immersed himself in the works of the great philosophers—Plato's *Republic,* Aristotle's *Organon,* Spi-noza's *Ethics,* Schopenhauer's *The World as Will and Idea.* He de-lighted in the good-natured teasing of his older sister about

Schopenhauer's deflated opinion of women. Though Sylvia was his confidante, the great minds of Socrates, Kant, and Descartes were his source of intellectual nourishment. Sylvia always believed that Bernard could have become a philosopher himself if events in his life had been different.

The stock market crash of 1929 and the ensuing Great Depression did not spare the Friedman family. Jacob's manufacturing business collapsed, and the family was forced to rent out their house in the Bronx in order to survive. Jacob stayed in New York and found work in the garment district, but the family moved to New Salem, Pennsylvania, where they lived with relatives on a small farm. Later they lived on the second floor of a grocery store that Sophie ran. The move was hard on the Friedman children. With no friends to speak of, Sylvia and Bernard became even closer. During the two years they stayed in Pennsylvania, they were constant companions.

Jacob's goal back in New York was to rebuild his business in dress manufacturing. When he visited the family in Pennsylvania, he brought dresses with him and enlisted Sylvia and Bernard to help him sell them. They loaded up the car and drove to nearby coal mines where they found buyers among the miners' wives who had no access to retail shops outside the company store.

Sylvia's contact with the Pennsylvania coal miners left a strong impression on her. She was moved by their struggle to survive the tough times of the depression. Years later she would draw upon her exposure to these families to help her understand and empathize with the obstacles faced by common people in their will to survive. Her understanding would serve her well in a struggle of a far different but equally daunting nature.

The depression was hard on the Friedman family, particularly on Sophie. Saddled with her own psychological depression, Sophie sometimes found herself having to choose between feeding herself or feeding her children. She always chose the latter, and Sylvia could see how stressful it was for her. A few years later her depression became so severe that she was placed in a sanitarium.

By this time the family had moved back to New York. With Sophie absent, Jacob felt pressed to send the children to live with relatives. But Sylvia again took charge. Though psychiatrists said her mother was in no condition to leave the hospital, Sylvia pressed for her release. "I'd like to have the chance to care for her," she told them. "I think she'll do better in her home environment surrounded by the family she loves. Just give me a chance."

Sylvia desperately wanted the family to stay together while also giving Sophie the strength and care to help her recover more quickly. Sylvia finally won out, her mother came home, and at age fifteen Sylvia continued as the family's primary caregiver. She prepared meals, did the shopping and, with Bernard's help, took charge of the laundry and housekeeping. She continued her education in high school but had to attend classes at night after her father returned home from a long day of work. It was a strenuous, difficult time for a young woman, but Sylvia was determined that the family would survive and remain together. "Mother did get better, but there was always the fear of a relapse, so I tried to keep her life as stress-free as possible," Sylvia recalled.

As emotionally draining as that period of Sylvia's life was, it built within her a rock-solid confidence. She felt that she could manage any situation. While still a teenager she had met the difficult circumstances of her mother's illness and carried the weight of running a household and overseeing a family, and it strengthened her. It prepared her for the challenges that lay ahead, the hardships and misfortunes.

3

BERNARD FRIEDMAN was the kind of son any mother would adore. He was bright, scholarly, and athletic. He and Sylvia spent hours hitting tennis balls to one another in the driveway of their home. Bernard taught her to hit a backhand and an overhand serve. He was the star of playground games, the first one chosen in pickup baseball games. His skill transferred to Sylvia. "He always insisted that I be selected on his team, even though I certainly wasn't as good a player as he was. His participation was conditional on having me accepted as a member of the team," she said.

For someone like Bernard—with so much physical prowess and such an enjoyment of sports—a serious illness seemed a particularly cruel fate. In 1937, Bernard was twenty-one years old, and a chronic disease was the last thing he expected to enter his life. He had experienced random symptoms for more than a year before he was formally diagnosed with MS. One morning he awoke and began seeing double as he tried to focus on the window in his bedroom. "I saw two tassels on the window shades, not the one that's there," he told Sylvia.

When this double vision persisted for several days, he went to an ophthalmologist who prescribed glasses and eye drops. The visual problems disappeared—a common phenomenon because of the transient nature of MS symptoms—and he returned to a normal life, at least for a while.

Soon thereafter Bernard started feeling pins-and-needles sensations in his legs and torso. Although the tingling was annoying and worrisome, the symptoms subsided as quickly as they had appeared. Bernard convinced himself that they were just a passing occurrence, and he put them out of his mind. But the symptoms recurred, each cycle more severe than the last. He also began to experience poor coordination and fatigue. Sylvia's concern about her brother's condition soon turned to anguish, and finally Bernard agreed to see one of New York's leading neurosurgeons. He conducted a series of tests, took x-rays, and poked Bernard with needles. He ruled out one disorder after another, from brain tumors to arthritis. Finally, with Bernard and Sylvia sitting across the desk from him, he gave them his diagnosis: multiple sclerosis.

The two of them were silent for a moment. "What's multiple sclerosis?" Sylvia finally asked. She had never heard of the disease.

The neurosurgeon explained MS to them. It was a rare disease of the central nervous system, he said, and only a few people had ever had it. He went on to explain that people with MS experienced attacks that could last for weeks or months, and in many cases their symptoms might diminish or disappear, only to resurface and perhaps intensify. Typical symptoms were impaired vision, numbness, and weakness. Some suffered tremors, an unsteady gait, even paralysis.

As his words sunk in, Sylvia and Bernard sat stunned. Then Sylvia asked, "What treatments can Bernard begin taking?"

The doctor offered no false hope. "There is really nothing that can be done for multiple sclerosis," he said. "We have no treatments. We have no cure. We don't even know what causes it. Bernard, about the only advice I can give you is to take it easy and rest. Don't be too active."

"What's his prognosis? What does the future hold?" Sylvia asked.

The doctor paused for a moment, then he looked directly at Bernard. "I'm not going to kid you. Your future is not hopeful, Bernard. You'll be fortunate to live five years with this ailment. That's the most I can promise you."

The doctor's sentence of death overwhelmed them both. Bernard was so distressed that he lost his bladder control and urinated on the doctor's expensive carpeting. The doctor was furious. "Get out of my office!" he shouted. "Both of you. That's all for today. Goodbye!" Then he abruptly ushered Bernard and Sylvia out the door and slammed it behind them.

The two were distraught. "Being diagnosed with a chronic disease like MS is frightening enough," Sylvia said. "But to be told that there were only a handful of other people who had the disease, and that there was no hope, made it all the more devastating."

Their experience was not unique, however. Other families coping with an MS diagnosis had similar traumas, though doctors did not always project such a dire future. Medical literature on MS at the time presented a bleak picture, yet the disease was not as rare as Sylvia and Bernard were told. Many doctors actually advised withholding the diagnosis from patients, calculating that knowledge of the disease and its hopelessness would only do them more harm. Many people with MS at the time found out about their disease only by accident, overhearing conversations of family members or inadvertently seeing a physician's notes. Relatives were told to keep the diagnosis a secret on the assumption that the truth would be too emotionally painful. In the view of many doctors, the reality of multiple sclerosis was worse than the unknown.

After they were so bluntly informed of Bernard's condition, Sylvia was unwilling to concede defeat. "Someone, somewhere, must know how to treat this disease," she said. They began searching for a doctor who might have a cure, or, at the very least, more knowledge. Most neurologists concurred with the first doctor's prognosis and provided Bernard with little hope. Finally they came upon a neurologist who refused to confirm Bernard's five-year life expectancy. "That hasn't been my experience with MS," he said. "It's an unpredictable disease. No one can say for certain how the course of the disease will evolve."

That statement provided Sylvia with a glimmer of hope, and it motivated her to search for other pieces of information that might breathe new life into Bernard's perspective on his future. At the time she was enrolled at Hunter College, studying English and business and aspiring to a career in law. But her concern for Bernard drove her to spend long hours in the medical library at the New York Academy of Medicine on Fifth Avenue in Manhattan, trying to learn all she could about MS. At the same time Bernard was doing his own research. Both of them found little. Most textbooks for general practitioners devoted no more than a paragraph or two to the disease. Journal articles on MS raised more questions than they answered, and offered little concrete information about the cause and even less about treatments.

Multiple sclerosis at that time was identified as an inflammatory disease of the central nervous system. Researchers knew that in people with MS, the myelin that surrounds the central nervous system fibers was lost in multiple areas. But for every piece of concrete knowledge there were a dozen unanswered questions. There were no reliable diagnostic standards for MS. There had been no viral or epidemiological studies. Immunology was still in its infancy. Meaningful treatments did not exist.

Yet there was no scarcity of theories about the underlying cause of MS. Some doctors erroneously believed that multiple sclerosis was triggered by a bacterial infection of spirochetes in the spinal fluid. Others believed it was caused by poisoning with metallic substances such as lead, mercury found in dental amalgam, arsenic, and tin. Others blamed allergic reactions manifesting themselves internally in the brain or the spinal cord. Sluggish blood flow in parts of the central nervous system was cited along with diets high in animal fat or diets deficient in vitamins.

Treatments ran the gamut from practical to outrageous. Some doctors tried to treat MS with antiseptics containing arsenic, mercury, and bismuth in hopes of combating infections that might be related to the disease. Fever therapy was used to burn away infectious agents. Anti-coagulant drugs such as heparin, or blood-vessel-dilating medications such as histamine and nicotinic acid, were administered to improve blood circulation. Anti-viral and anti-allergy medications were widely used. High doses of every kind of vitamin were prescribed, and all kinds of diets from low-fat to gluten-free to fish-oil-rich were recommended. Other physicians resorted to psychiatric care, hypnosis, tonsillectomies, and tooth extractions. In Russia, vaccines were created from viruses supposedly taken from the brains of people with MS. All of these approaches had their true believers; none produced verifiable cures. Reputable doctors gradually abandoned them, leaving MS sufferers and their families discouraged and despondent.

Bernard and Sylvia waded through the textbooks as best they could, often with a medical dictionary at their sides. Though their findings provided little more than a bleak outlook for Bernard, they were touched and inspired by the sincerity they found in the writings of several neurologists who cared for people with MS. Wrote Dr. Richard Brickner of New York's Mt. Sinai Hospital, "Although I've never had multiple sclerosis, I suffer from it."

For his part, Bernard wrote letters to neurologists at the country's leading medical centers—Johns Hopkins, the Mayo Clinic, New York University, and many others. The replies were universally discouraging: there are no proven therapies for MS, the course of MS is unpredictable, but for most people with the disease, there is a worsening of symptoms, often leading to premature death. The responses were so consistently disheartening that Sylvia began intercepting the mail whenever she could in order to keep the letters from Bernard's eyes. She felt she had to lift his spirits even if it meant shielding him from the potentially devastating nature of his disease. She was to continue this protective nature for decades as Bernard fought his illness.

At one point Bernard declared, "I've got to work hard to earn money that I can set aside for the time when I'll be totally disabled." He began working double time as production manager in his father's factory, which at that point was manufacturing venetian blinds. Yet he never amassed a nest egg, choosing instead to be paid only pocket money because he felt the family needed the money more than he did.

As the months and years passed, Bernard's health gradually began to take more of an emotional toll on him and Sylvia.

They felt anger, sadness, and depression. "Bernie was not only my brother, he was my closest friend," Sylvia said. His well-being became her top priority. She put her own dreams on hold, deciding that the defeat of multiple sclerosis would be her life's work.

4

FROM THE EARLIEST DAYS of her brother's battle with multiple sclerosis, Sylvia Friedman believed that a cure for his illness would be discovered. She constantly shared that dream with Bernard and the rest of the family. She was determined to keep their spirits high, even though she felt frustrated and frightened.

Although Sylvia had told her parents about Bernard's diagnosis, she protected them from the gloomy scenario offered by the New York neurosurgeon who had given Bernard just five years to live at the optimum. Her mother and father had never heard of MS, and they were unaware of the seriousness of Bernard's illness. Sylvia insisted on protecting her mother in particular, since doctors believed that stress could trigger a recurrence of her depression.

It was now the early 1940s, the nation was at war, and Sylvia tried to instill a sense of normalcy in her own life. She managed a law office and became a hearing reporter for the U.S. attorney's office. Her job was to take testimony largely from members of the German-American Bund, as part of the war effort.

She met her future husband, and when they married in 1943 she became Sylvia Lawry, and they moved into an apartment. Bernard, meanwhile, continued to live with his parents and younger sisters. Sylvia went through a Red Cross training course for nurses' aides and volunteered at New York's St. Clare's Hospital. Even though she had a very busy life, she never stopped worrying about Bernard and tending to his needs. They remained extremely close. "When I was a teenager I had assumed the responsibility for bringing up my siblings, and I felt like the head of the family," she said. "So I continued to feel responsible for Bernard and his well-being."

Bernard began undergoing a number of experimental treatments recommended by a neurologist. None had encouraging track records, but Bernard was willing to try these therapies in the hope that one of them might work. At one point he was inoculated with the bacteria that caused typhoid. Though a potentially life-threatening treatment, it was touted as a possible cure for MS. Because typhoid causes the body temperature to rise to very high levels, the theory was that the fever could burn out the spirochetes or other organisms that might be the cause of MS. Over a period of several days Bernard received several injections which raised his temperature high enough to leave him bedridden. The MS persisted, however, and the treatment was considered a failure.

Bernard tried other approaches. He took vitamins. He consumed wheat germ. Nothing helped. He continued to have an exacerbation every year, and his condition progressively worsened. In the war years, thousands of doctors had become part of the armed forces. During 1943–1944, approximately one-third of America's physicians were in the service. This placed a huge burden on those doctors who remained at home. There were not only fewer doctors available to care for people with MS, but there was a virtual halt to most studies of the disease. The research that went on was piecemeal and un-coordinated. For MS patients like Bernard, many of whom experienced a worsening of their disease with time, the war years were particularly and personally devastating.

Nevertheless Bernard did find a neurologist whom he liked and trusted. Whenever new symptoms developed, Sylvia and Bernard would routinely see this doctor. After a number of these visits, however, Sylvia was stunned when Bernard was refused another appointment. The doctor told her, "If Bernard has a severe attack that puts him in a crisis situation, I'll see him. But there's nothing I can do for him, so it's a waste of everyone's time for me to examine him routinely."

Despite his illness, Bernard continued to live as normal a life as possible. In 1942 he went to Florida on vacation and met a young woman. There was instant chemistry between them, and before he returned to New York she invited him to meet her parents. The families thought a marriage might be in the works. But once Bernard came home, he never made an effort to get in touch with the young woman again. She wrote him letters which he left unanswered. "Bernie truly believed what doctors had told him, that he didn't have much hope of a long life," Sylvia recalled. "So at the time, marriage was out of the question. He didn't think it was fair to pursue a relationship with this woman. So he just let it go."

As Bernard's illness continued to progress, so did Sylvia's concern for his well-being. He developed problems walking, and she worried about his safety while maneuvering through traffic to get to his job at their father's factory.

Then one evening she received an alarming phone call from one of her sisters. "We found a suicide note that Bernie wrote," she said. "In the note he says that he's prepared to kill himself, although he doesn't say when or how. Sylvia, he's just given up on life."

Sylvia's husband Michael Lawry, whom she had married in 1944, insisted that they bring Bernard to live with them. "You'll worry less if Bernie's in our home," he said. "We can keep a close eye on him and make sure he's okay."

But there wasn't enough room in their small apartment to accommodate Bernard, so Sylvia's parents purchased a home in the country where Bernard could live with Sylvia and her husband. Bernard stopped working at his father's plant, and by living away from high-traffic areas he could take walks safely. He also did not have daily contact with his mother, who was always at risk of another breakdown. "I knew if she watched Bernie go downhill, it would destroy her," Sylvia said.

Sylvia even quit her job in order to take care of Bernard. "My husband loved my brother very much," she said. "It was no burden to him to have Bernie live with us. And it made me less anxious. So Bernie began a very sedentary existence in our home."

Sylvia, however, could scarcely remain sedentary with regard to her brother's illness. The horror of his suicide note haunted her, and she felt that she had to do something more to find help. She continued to read everything she could about MS, but there seemed to be nothing close to a breakthrough in finding a cure. "If I could find just one person who has experienced a remission of MS," she told herself, "that individual might have an idea of what brought that remission about. And we could try that treatment on Bernie."

That is when she had the idea of running the classified ad in the *New York Times*. She simply wanted to hear from someone who had recovered from MS. The advertising staff at the *Times* at first declined to run the ad. They wanted more information

about who Sylvia was, fearing that she might be a quack looking for gullible people with MS. Finally the ad appeared. She
was assigned box #272 at the *Times* office, and she eagerly
awaited correspondence. She had no idea at the time that she
was about to embark on a long, arduous journey in the fight
against her brother's disease. There had never been an organized campaign against MS, and launching such an effort was
not even a consideration. She had placed the ad for the sake of
Bernard, and perhaps for the sake of others with MS.

Little did she know what she had started.

5

IN THE WAKE of World War II, most Americans could feel a sense of increased optimism about their health. With funds no longer needed for the war effort, the federal government launched its most aggressive financing of biomedical research ever, mobilized by Congress's enactment of the Public Health Service Act. The National Institutes of Health increased its research grants tenfold, from $85,000 in 1945 to $850,000 in 1946. Most of these dollars were directed into laboratories at major universities and medical schools, where studies were launched that would lead to one major breakthrough after another, from new immunizations to organ transplantation. Even so, multiple sclerosis remained an overlooked, neglected orphan among diseases. While organizations like the American Heart Association and the American Cancer Society were flexing their muscles to make certain that research funds were directed into the study of their respective diseases, no one was speaking out on behalf of people with MS. There was nowhere for MS families to turn for answers, and little reason for genuine hope.

Still, Sylvia and Bernard believed that perhaps a cure for his illness would be found in the responses to the classified ad that she had placed in the *New York Times*. Perhaps an MS patient had found a drug, developed a diet, or adopted a regimen of physical therapy that had turned MS around and that could also help Bernard.

In fact, nearly all the letters responding to the ad were from people with MS, or their family members, who were much like Bernard and Sylvia. They too were desperate for anything that might cure or at least halt the progression of the disease. They shared a common anguish, the same frustration. And almost every one of them conveyed the same message: "If you find out anything about MS treatments, please let us know."

One letter, however, was different. It was unsigned. It had no return address, though it carried a Philadelphia postmark. The writer claimed that his wife had been cured of MS by a European neurologist named Otto Marburg. He explained that his spouse had been diagnosed with MS twenty-five years earlier. "She became completely paralyzed," the letter writer said. "But all of her MS symptoms vanished after Dr. Marburg treated her. She recovered completely, and has had no recurrences."

Sylvia read and reread the letter. In explaining why he had chosen anonymity, the letter writer said that his wife had never been told of her MS diagnosis, and he did not want to take a chance that any communication about her medical condition might reach her. He added that Dr. Marburg had left Europe and was now practicing medicine at the Neurological Institute in New York City.

"This is the information we're looking for," Sylvia told her brother excitedly.

With their expectations soaring, they made an appointment to see Dr. Marburg, hoping that he could provide Bernard with treatment that could stop his disease in its tracks.

Otto Marburg was an Austrian-born neurologist who was recognized throughout Europe, primarily for his work in epilepsy and brain tumors. After fleeing to America as a refugee from the Nazis, he joined the staff of the Neurological Institute at the College of Physicians and Surgeons of Columbia University. When Sylvia and Bernard arrived in his office, she showed him the letter from Philadelphia. Marburg scanned it quickly and said, "I know who this person is, and I recall exactly how I treated his wife. I'll prescribe the same treatment for Bernard. It's called nicotinic acid. It's a B vitamin that historically has been used to prevent a disease called pellagra. Nicotinic acid is a vasodilator, and I've found that it helps some people with MS, but not others. So I can't guarantee how successful it will be for your brother. But we can try it."

Bernard was eager to put nicotinic acid to the test. Sylvia, who had begun to correspond with some of the people who had answered the *Times* ad, told other MS families about her meeting with Dr. Marburg—and about the patient in Philadelphia who had become symptom-free—and it gave them hope too.

Bernard began Dr. Marburg's treatment, but after several weeks his condition did not improve. It was a terrible disappointment. As both Bernard and Sylvia agonized over the treatment failure, she wondered how many more setbacks he could withstand. At the same time she began contemplating what her next move would be.

At about this time, Sylvia suggested that the respondents to her *Times* ad meet one another. About a dozen of them started getting together regularly in a meeting room donated by the Red Cross in Brooklyn. They shared their MS experiences and discussed the search for possible solutions. There was Victor

Young, an engineer who first became aware of his illness when he tumbled down a flight of stairs in Penn Station. John Freund, a reporter for the *New York Daily News,* believed that drinking grape juice had allowed him to remain active for years after his diagnosis. Others spoke of experiencing bouts of incredible fatigue, unexplainable weakness in their legs, and even being sent to psychiatrists after being told that there was "nothing wrong" with their bodies. They leaned on one another for support, and at times they shed tears together. Also, beginning at their first meeting, they began to discuss the possibility of creating an organization to support research into MS. The seeds had been planted.

For Sylvia, a woman just thirty years old, the challenge of launching an organized movement to seek a cure for a disease unfamiliar to most Americans seemed an impossible undertaking. Were Bernard not so seriously ill, she might not have pursued it. "I felt it was something I had to do," she said, "even though I wasn't sure where it would lead."

Meanwhile Sylvia resumed her research in the medical library. She read of dramatic breakthroughs with other diseases. Scarlet fever was being treated successfully with penicillin. New antibiotics, including streptomycin, had been introduced. A cure for cholera, once a devastating plague, was developed. But of the scant number of significant articles about MS, none signaled a breakthrough on the horizon.

In her reading, however, she repeatedly came across the name of Dr. Tracy Putnam, director of the Neurological Institute of New York. Dr. Putnam seemed to have a special interest in MS, and Sylvia decided to approach him with her idea of launching a society devoted to MS research. With her sister Alice, Sylvia met with Dr. Putnam in his office. He was a dignified, Harvard-educated physician with a pleasant smile and a reputation for showing great compassion for his patients.

"We're interested in stimulating research into MS," Sylvia began. "Do you feel there is sufficient interest in the medical community to warrant such an effort on our part?"

Dr. Putnam paused for a moment, then pointed to a $25 check on his desk. It was a donation from a family affected by multiple sclerosis. They were among many with whom Dr. Putnam had been in touch, some of whom he treated at no cost. "I think I'm on the verge of a promising new development in MS," Dr. Putnam said. "But the board of directors at my hospital doesn't know anything about MS and hasn't offered financial support for my research. They're much more interested in diseases like cancer and polio that are getting so much public attention. So I'm struggling along with the pitiful contributions that come in. If an effective organization were developed, I believe more researchers would want to work in this field. I would certainly be interested in expanding my own research efforts."

Would he serve as chairman of a medical advisory board?

Dr. Putnam didn't hesitate. "I'll put together a list of prominent neurologists around the country whom you can invite to serve on your medical board. If they want me to serve as chairman, yes, I will," he said.

Sylvia was exhilarated by his response. She believed that if her efforts could put tools and technologies into the hands of dedicated researchers, a cure for MS might be within reach. A week later Dr. Putnam's list of neurologists was in her hands, and she began typing invitations to these doctors to participate on the board. All but one accepted. Sylvia had cleared the first major hurdle in her effort to start an MS organization.

In March 1946, with Dr. Putnam and several other leading

neurologists on board, Sylvia persuaded attorney Irving Berkelhammer to draw up papers of incorporation for the organization. Berkelhammer had responded to her ad in the *Times*
because his brother, a dentist, had MS. Once the documents
were prepared and signed, the society was formally created
under the name Association for the Advancement of Research
on Multiple Sclerosis.

The new organization had four basic missions:

—Coordinate research efforts on multiple sclerosis in this
country and abroad.

—Gather statistics on the prevalence and geographical distribution of MS.

—Act as a clearinghouse for information on this disease.

—Collect funds to stimulate and support research on MS
and allied diseases.

The framework was straightforward, the motive sincere,
the goal uncomplicated.

"I really had no idea what I was getting into," Sylvia said.
"At the time it seemed like a simple undertaking—to raise
enough money to support significant research projects. Our intent was to spend 100 percent of the money we raised on research. But I thought the path would be a much easier one
than it turned out to be. I really believed this would be a short-
term undertaking. Of course, I was wrong."

Sylvia convinced officials at the Academy of Medicine to
donate a one-room, eight-by-ten-foot office at its headquarters
at Fifth Avenue and 103rd Street in New York. "I had been in
the Academy's building, reading medical books, and saw that
there was an empty office," Sylvia recalled. "I figured it would
be a prestigious address for us. So I asked for the office as a donation. It's amazing how far you can get just by asking."

The office seemed more like a walk-in closet, requiring a

shoehorn to get into and out of. But it fit the association's needs in those early days.

The next step, Sylvia felt, was to issue a press release announcing the formation of the new organization. As she worked on a first draft, John Freund offered to introduce her to Waldemar Kaempffert, the science editor of the *New York Times*. "I think he can guide you on the writing of that release." Sylvia met with Kaempffert at his office at the *Times*, holding the draft of her press release in her hand. He had been the newspaper's science editor for almost twenty years and wrote a popular weekly column that had elevated him to the stature of one of journalism's leading interpreters of medical and scientific information. Sylvia told him what she had: the skeleton of a new organization, a medical advisory board, a small group of persons with MS and their families with whom she had been meeting, and huge hopes for the future.

Kaempffert read the first draft of her press release, then offered some advice. "I wouldn't issue this yet," he told her. "Before you do, you need to recruit a board of directors from the power structure of the nation—people whose names can create public confidence in the organization and get attention from the press."

Although Kaempffert's suggestion made sense, Sylvia hardly knew where to begin. She decided to take a job in the New York mayoral campaign of William O'Dwyer, motivated solely by the need to meet prominent, influential people whom she might convince to lend their names to the new association. Running the campaign's speakers' bureau, she met and began to interest the power brokers in O'Dwyer's coterie. But none of them impressed Kaempffert. "Go after nationally known figures," he insisted. She found, however, that most of the people she approached had never heard of multiple sclerosis. When she told them that doctors believed it was a rare disease, they immediately lost interest.

Her frustration nearly turned to despair. Would the organization collapse almost before it began? Despite her disappointments, however, Sylvia wasn't willing to quit. Again Dr. Putnam opened an important door for her.

Putnam was becoming uneasy. Months had passed since his initial meeting with Sylvia. Whenever they spoke, he could sense her increasing dejection over the snail's pace at which the association was developing. That changed one afternoon when he called her from his office.

"Mrs. Lawry, I'd like you to meet the father of an MS patient whom I've just diagnosed. He's extremely well placed and wealthy. I told him that a foundation for MS had been set up, and I asked if he'd like to learn more about it. He said that he'd be willing to meet with you," Putnam said. The man was Otto Frohnknecht. He was founder and chairman of the board of the International Minerals and Metals Corporation. Frohnknecht was very much a businessman, yet both of his daughters had married artists—author/playwright Arthur Kober and conductor Erich Leinsdorf. According to Dr. Putnam, Frohnknecht was devastated when his daughter, Margaret Kober, was diagnosed with MS. He was looking for somewhere to turn to deal with the reality that she had a disease with no known cause or cure—and where research appeared to be the only solution.

Sylvia met with Frohnknecht in his elegant office and described the slow pace at which she was forming a board of directors. Once the board was in place, she said, the association planned to move ahead with the funding of research.

"How much money does your association presently have in the bank?" Frohnknecht asked.

A bit embarrassed, Sylvia replied, "About $5,000." It was money she herself had contributed, along with funds from some of the people who had responded to her ad in the *Times*.

"Oh, my God!" Frohnknecht said. "$5,000!" His face fell. Then he asked, "Why should I put money into your Society instead of making a direct contribution to Dr. Putnam or another scientist doing research?"

"An organization can multiply the benefits received from any single contribution," Sylvia answered. "If you contribute to us, we can build upon it, using it to encourage others to make contributions. We plan to establish a research fund in which 100 percent of our contributions will go to research grants. None of it will be spent on administrative costs."

Frohnknecht reached for his checkbook in a desk drawer, wrote out a contribution of $1,000, and handed it to her. "If you know how to spend that, there will be more to come," he said.

Frohnknecht called the next day. "Mrs. Lawry, I think you ought to meet with my lawyer, who is also a friend of mine," he said. "He might help develop your foundation. He has excellent contacts and would know how best to proceed."

The lawyer, Carl M. Owen, headed one of New York's most prestigious law firms and specialized in corporate law. One of his law partners was Wendell Willkie, who had been defeated by Franklin Roosevelt in the 1940 presidential election. Owen was routinely in contact with the who's who of business, society, and culture in New York and the country.

Sylvia met Owen under very unusual circumstances—so unusual, in fact, that she wondered whether the first impression she made would undermine whatever hope she had of recruiting Owen to the cause. Frohnknecht had arranged the meeting in Owen's office on Wall Street, and Sylvia had arrived

early and had had breakfast in a nearby restaurant. As the wait-
ress was refilling her coffee cup, the coffee splashed on Sylvia's
dress. "I was stunned," Sylvia recalled. "There wasn't enough
time to buy a dress and change, and I debated whether to cancel the meeting. Finally I decided to go through with it. I
walked into Carl's office and jokingly pointed to my dress. We
both had a good laugh. He enjoyed that unusual introduction
quite a bit."

Owen's first effort was to reach out to Basil O'Connor, a
former classmate of Owen's at the Harvard Law School, and
convince him to meet with Sylvia. O'Connor was a Wall Street
lawyer who had become the driving force behind the foundation supporting polio research. He was just the person Sylvia
wanted to meet. Otto Frohnknecht had suggested that perhaps
O'Connor would be willing to take multiple sclerosis under the
Polio Foundation's wing as part of its mission.

At the time no disease in America had a higher profile
than polio. Polio epidemics were ravaging thousands of lives
and prompting anxious parents to keep their children away
from crowds by forbidding them to use public swimming pools
and to go to movie theaters. Through its March of Dimes campaign, the National Foundation for Infantile Paralysis was raising millions of dimes a year that were funneled into research by
Dr. Jonas Salk and others. "Perhaps some of that money could
be spent on MS," Frohnknecht said.

Carl Owen arranged a meeting with Sylvia and O'Connor,
who had already served for eight years as president of the National Foundation. O'Connor had dedicated thousands of
hours to the fight against polio. He had told friends that he
made the commitment to infantile paralysis after seeing
Franklin Roosevelt (who had polio) fall helplessly onto the
floor in the Manhattan office building where O'Connor had

his law practice. Over lunch, Sylvia proposed broadening the scope of the National Foundation to include MS. O'Connor asked for some time to think about it. A few days later he called and turned down her proposal. "If we took on MS, there's no reason to believe that we'd raise more money, and we're committed to spending our funds on solving the polio problem," he said. But then O'Connor added, "There can be a separate but equally strong foundation for multiple sclerosis. It's a very good cause. All that's needed is a strong organization."

O'Connor offered to provide Lawry with all the basic documents that the National Foundation had used—it's charter, constitution, bylaws, chapter manuals, and grant application forms. He also recommended that she set up two boards: a lay board of directors, with the power to make decisions and allocate funds; and a separate medical advisory board. He told her, "With a strong organization you can raise as much money as we do."

Shortly thereafter, with Otto Frohnknecht's approval, Sylvia decided to ask Carl Owen to become president of the new MS association. Owen declined, but he offered his help in organizing the board of prominent sponsors that she had been trying so hard to build. Owen didn't let her down. In corporate board rooms and on golf courses, he recruited his high-powered colleagues. They were devoted to him, and one after another they agreed to help. Mrs. Wendell L. Willkie came on board. So did U.S. Senator Brien McMahon; Harrison Tweed, president of the Bar Association of the City of New York; and Matthew Woll, vice president of the American Federation of Labor. Hugo Rogers, borough president of Manhattan, added his name to the list, as did Edgar Bolles, chairman of the board of the General Reinsurance Company, and John Rovensky, chairman of the American Car and Foundry Company. In all there were eleven names on the list, including Owen and Frohnknecht. They were an impressive, influential group, the kind that gave the new association the clout it would need to attract media attention.

Meanwhile the initial press release had gone through several more drafts. Sylvia wanted it just right. Not only did Kaempffert review it again and again, but so did journalists from the *New York Daily News,* the Associated Press, and the Scripps newspaper chain. Dr. Iago Galdston, director of public information at the Academy of Medicine, also read it.

Finally, on October 3, 1946, the press release was issued. It began, "Formation of an organization to fight a grave nerve disease, which cripples thousands yearly but about which little is known, was announced today." The release generated worldwide media attention. It was printed or excerpted by nearly every major newspaper and many magazines in the country. The *New York Times* published two articles—one in the Sunday *Times,* written by Waldemar Kaempffert, and the other in the daily paper, using the headline, "New Unit to Fight Crippling Malady." It quoted Dr. Galdston as saying, "For a long time there has been a crying need for just such an organization. . . . This new movement should help us to gain some light in a field where at present there is a great deal of darkness."

The press release gave multiple sclerosis the highest visibility it had ever enjoyed in the United States. The response to the many newspaper and magazine articles was overwhelming. Nearly ten thousand letters from around the world flooded into the organization's tiny Academy of Medicine office. Perhaps MS was not as rare as doctors and medical textbooks had claimed.

Not all of the feedback was positive, however. The day the *Times* article appeared, Sylvia received an angry phone call from a New York resident who shouted his way through their entire conversation. "It sounds like you're trying to get money from MS patients," he fumed. "Can't you just leave us alone instead of exploiting us? What's wrong with you people? What will doctors think of next?"

The man's vitriolic attack shook Sylvia. She had never been confronted with such anger. But she let the man talk. Finally she made a request that surprised him. "If you'll allow me, I'd like to meet with you to explain what the Association is all about." He quieted down momentarily, then invited her to his home. With some trepidation, she agreed to visit him the next day.

"When I arrived I found this paralyzed man with MS, living alone," Sylvia said. "He told me that he conducted an insurance business over the phone from his bed, and supported himself this way. In that sense he was quite remarkable, but he certainly made no friendly gestures at first. However, as I explained my dreams for the Society, and what we hoped to accomplish, I gradually began to win him over. In fact, before I left, he actually told me that he'd help in any way he could. Over the next few years he became one of our most active volunteers, and he recruited many new members for us."

Sylvia considered this tense encounter a watershed event in her life. Although she had been verbally assaulted, she refused to back off. She confronted her own fears and insecurities, and ultimately gained the support of a man who had been so defiant. It boosted her own self-confidence. And it convinced her that she had what it took to move the new organization forward.

6

CARL OWEN rarely shied away from a challenge. Born in Galena, Ohio, he earned his way through college at Dartmouth by selling Bibles door-to-door. At Harvard Law School he edited the prestigious *Law Review* and graduated summa cum laude. After he was admitted to the New York Bar in 1906, he became a partner in a law firm that, after two mergers, evolved into the prominent Willkie, Owen, Farr, Gallagher & Walton. He became one of Wendell Willkie's most trusted advisers, and when Willkie ran for the presidency in 1940, Owen frequently was by his side on the campaign trail.

Even so, Owen approached the MS Society with caution. When Sylvia Lawry asked him to become president of the new organization, he took a wait-and-see attitude. Until Otto Frohnknecht's daughter was diagnosed with MS, Owen had never heard of the disease. As impressed as he was with Sylvia's unwavering commitment, he was still uncertain about the future of the organization. Nevertheless Owen began giving more of his time to it.

After recruiting members of the board of sponsors, he met

with his clients in the advertising industry, who recommended that the Association place ads in newspapers in Boston. The ads would announce the creation of the new national organization for multiple sclerosis, and encourage communication from interested parties. Boston was chosen because of its growing reputation as a center of medical research and the hub of the neurological community, making it more likely that people with MS would be properly diagnosed there compared with other parts of the country. "The response will help us get a sense of just how widespread MS is," Owen told Sylvia. He felt that if the ads stimulated a sizable response, he'd feel justified in assuming the presidency of an organization dedicated to a largely unknown health problem.

The ads ran in the *Boston Globe* and the *Boston Herald* for just a day. But that was enough to stimulate an astonishing flood of mail into the association's tiny office. Letters arrived from physicians and scientists, wanting to know more about the organization and the research that it promised to support. Inquiries came from the families of individuals with multiple sclerosis. There were emotional pleas from people with MS, desperate for ways to cope with a chronic illness that was gradually taking over their bodies. Within ten days, five thousand letters had overrun Sylvia Lawry's desk. She was stunned by the response—and so was Carl Owen. He came into the office late one afternoon and saw boxes full of letters, all from Boston and surrounding communities, many of them not yet opened. He called Sylvia the next day and said, "I'd be honored to serve as your first president."

As 1946 drew to a close, Sylvia began planning the first meeting of the Medical Advisory Board of the Association for the Advancement of Research on Multiple Sclerosis. It was a logistical challenge pinning down a date when all of the board members—twenty of the nation's leading neurologists—would be available to gather in New York City. After a seemingly endless exchange of correspondence and phone calls, they finally agreed on a Friday evening in February 1947.

On the afternoon before the meeting, however, snow flurries began, followed by a snowstorm that struck New York with a vengeance. The storm blasted the city for more than thirty hours, creating one of the heaviest, most extraordinary snowfalls in its history. Streets were blanketed by more than a foot of snow. Although city crews operated dozens of snowplows around the clock, most roads remained hopelessly choked, with many cars and trucks abandoned in the streets. All of the eastern seaboard airports shut down for hours until the snow could be cleared from their runways.

Sylvia was frantic in the hours before the meeting. She had attached so many of her hopes to this crucial gathering. But now a blizzard had intervened, possibly sabotaging the meeting and perhaps many of Sylvia's dreams as well.

Her fears, however, were groundless. Although the storm was severe, nearly all the neurologists found their way into Manhattan for the meeting. They came from as far away as San Francisco, Montreal, and Rochester, Minnesota. Ironically, only Dr. Tracy Putnam, chairman of the Medical Advisory Board and a New Yorker himself, became hopelessly stranded in a snowbound airport and never reached the meeting room at the Academy of Medicine.

The scientists at that gathering were the most renowned figures in modern neurology, affiliated with the nation's most prestigious medical centers. Among them were Dr. Henry W. Woltman of the Mayo Clinic, Dr. Richard Brickner of the Neurological Institute in New York, and Dr. Francis Schwentker of Johns Hopkins Hospital. For hours they discussed current theories about the causes of multiple sclerosis and therapies that might be developed. Dr. Gabriel Steiner of the Wayne State University College of Medicine conjectured that the coiled bacterium called a spirochete—perhaps related to the same family of organisms that triggers syphilis and relapsing fever—might play a role in MS. Dr. Thomas Rivers of the Rockefeller Institute for Medical Research, which had become the center for viral research in the United States, described his own skepticism that a virus played a role in MS.

Dr. Putnam had prepared a paper to present to the panel. In his absence Carl Owen read it to the assembled neurologists. "MS is gradually becoming recognized as one of the most baffling and devastating diseases, claiming thousands of victims all over the world each year," Dr. Putnam wrote. "Many authorities have observed that the original onset of the disease has been precipitated by such factors as infections of the respiratory tract, pneumonia, overexertion, exposure to cold, shock, poisoning, and pregnancy. The disease flourishes in cold, damp climates and is rare in warm, dry climates."

As Sylvia Lawry had predicted, the meeting was an intellectually stimulating forum. Nevertheless she left that night feeling bitterly disappointed. "These doctors were the recognized leaders in neurology, and all of them had a known interest in MS," she said. "Up until the meeting itself, I had thought that by giving these great minds a venue to talk among themselves, something dramatic and exciting would be revealed. I had believed that the real problem was a lack of communication about what was known about MS—only to realize that very little was known about it. That's how naive I was."

The neurologists reacted quite differently. Many returned home feeling a sense of relief. Better than anyone, they understood that the causes of multiple sclerosis were unknown and that no treatment had survived the test of time. But with the new MS association there was finally an organized campaign to fund research into this puzzling disease. They no longer felt that they were drifting aimlessly at sea. As Dr. Putnam had written in his paper, neurologists had believed for many years that there was a need for a program of intensive research into MS; with the new association, he said, the promise of that kind of program was finally in place.

Carl Owen also was encouraged by what he heard that night. One of his goals for the meeting was to determine the degree of genuine interest that existed among those who had agreed to serve on the Medical Advisory Board. Was the board merely window dressing, or was it the nucleus of a real participatory body? Through the give and take of the board members that night, and the sense of commitment they showed, Owen got the answer he wanted.

In the days that followed, Sylvia was buoyed by great hope—but weighed down with the enormous responsibility upon her shoulders. The avalanche of mail and phone calls continued. Desperate people sought information about any new treatment that might arrest the progression of their illness. Some pleaded for services that didn't exist. Sylvia worked fourteen- and fifteen-hour days—but a one-woman operation could not keep up with the demands. The association's membership rolls, which began with those first few people who had answered the *Times* ad in 1945, was steadily growing, but its bank account remained modest. There never seemed to be enough funds to cover more than the barest of expenses. While other voluntary health agencies conducted fundraising campaigns among the public, often with help of a network of chapters, the MS movement had no manpower at the local level. It relied on modest $3 dues from members, many of whom were recruited by existing members, or who joined after contacting the Association for information about the disease. People who couldn't afford the dues were given a complimentary membership.

Meanwhile, Sylvia could only look at other health agencies with envy. The National Foundation for Infantile Paralysis raised money through collection boxes placed in thousands of movie theaters across the country, and it could rely on the support of Hollywood stars such as Helen Hayes and Marlene Dietrich, both of whom had children with polio. The American Cancer Society, which had once been a physician-dominated organization, was transformed into a voluntary health association with the help of a nationwide legion of volunteers—the so-called Women's Field Army—who collected more than $10 million in 1946. By contrast, the MS organization's entire first-year projected budget was $10,000, and at one point Sylvia wondered where those funds would come from. Then Otto Frohnknecht agreed to underwrite $5,000, and a New York diamond merchant named Alexander Arnstein, who had MS, pledged $5,000. But Sylvia was able to raise $10,000 from small contributors, so she didn't have to call on the two $5,000 pledges; those generous contributions were made anyway.

Sylvia and Carl Owen were volunteers, drawing no salary and feeling their way during those early months. Owen told her, "You have to crawl before you learn to walk. Through adversity, you become stronger than if everything comes easy." Maybe so, Sylvia said. But during those late nights in the office, as she answered mail and hoped for a miracle, she would have preferred an easier path.

"I rarely had a moment to come up for air," she said. "But I also felt encouraged knowing that after years of frustration when Bernard and I had followed the will-o'-the-wisps of new therapies, none of which got him anywhere, I was finally doing something positive that might produce a real breakthrough."

As she read the mail on her desk, however, and recognized the enormous unmet need for MS-related education, research, and rehabilitation programs, she felt overwhelmed. She often spent the entire night at her desk sustained by only a percolating coffee pot and the determination to persevere.

7

———

I F SYLVIA LAWRY ever questioned the need for a national society dedicated to multiple sclerosis, those doubts vanished
when the new organization began holding meetings for its
members in a theater-sized auditorium at the New York Academy of Medicine.

From the start, these monthly meetings attracted standing-
room-only crowds. On the one hand, it was a social evening in
which people with MS and their families could interact with
others living with the disease, sharing experiences and providing support. But there was a more serious side to the gatherings. Each month Lawry invited neurologists to speak on a
relevant topic and answer questions. For the first time many MS
families had a source of reliable information about the disease.
She encouraged the doctors to emphasize the positive while
still being realistic about the course of the illness.

As word of the meetings grew, people came from all parts
of New York City, New Jersey, Connecticut, and even farther
away. Some arrived in wheelchairs. Others showed no signs of
their disease. "People were excited about what we were doing,"

said Sylvia, "and they wanted to stay in touch." As they understood more about the disease, they often experienced some relief from the anxiety and despair that so often accompanies a
diagnosis of multiple sclerosis.

The crowds might have been even larger if more doctors
had been honest with their patients. It continued to be a time
when the diagnosis of multiple sclerosis was often hidden from
people with the disease. Some physicians even discouraged
Sylvia from launching a society devoted to MS. When she met
with Israel Straus, a leading New York neurologist, in his West
59th Street office, she asked him to let his patients with MS
know of the existence of the new organization.

Dr. Straus was indignant. "I don't think people with MS
should be told their diagnosis!" he said. "Most just can't cope
with it." As he led her to the door, he added, "If this Society gets
off the ground, you'll be opening up a Pandora's box. You'll
find that the needs of individuals with MS are so enormous that
you won't be able to handle it. You better think again about
what you're doing."

Sylvia's next challenge was to assemble a lay board of directors—a group that would replace the original board members who had initially lent their names to the cause. She wanted
to attract people whose families had been touched by MS. Just
as significantly, she wanted people with connections that could
help the organization in its growth and fundraising.

Sylvia spoke with a member of the Medical Advisory Board
whose prestigious medical center attracted people with MS
from across the country for consultations about their illness.
He agreed with her approach and confidentially gave Sylvia the
names of many prominent families who had been affected by
MS. She arranged for introductions to these individuals, without ever revealing her source of the information that the dis-

ease was in their families, and pleaded her case. "This organization offers people with MS their best hope for a cure," she told them. "If you won't support us, who will?"

The lay board was formed in 1946 and 1947. Ten of the eighteen members were connected to MS in this direct way. They were an impressive, diverse body. They included Alida Camp, whose husband Frederic, dean of the Stevens Institute of Technology, was an MS patient; Ralph I. Straus, director of R. H. Macy and Company, whose mother had MS; Henry J. Kaiser, Jr., who had MS and was the son of the famed industrialist; and William C. Breed, Jr., a partner in the prominent New York law firm Breed, Abbott & Morgan, who had a brother with MS. From the beginning, it was an active, working board, and it would remain that way for more than fifty years.

As Sylvia Lawry opened the stack of mail on her desk one morning, one letter in particular caught her attention. It had been written by Raymond Moley, and she immediately recognized his name. Anyone who paid attention to the administration of Franklin Roosevelt knew of Moley, who had been a member of FDR's Brain Trust. He was one of the leading architects of Roosevelt's depression-fighting programs; in 1933 he had coined the term "New Deal." By the end of Roosevelt's first term, however, Moley had left FDR's inner circle, and shortly thereafter he became a columnist and contributing editor at *Newsweek*. He eventually threw his support to Wendell Willkie in the Republican candidate's 1940 campaign against Roosevelt. In Moley's letter he requested literature about MS and included a $50 donation to the Society, which in those days was a large contribution. His national stature, however, was what most interested Sylvia. She called and asked to meet with him.

"When I was a professor at Barnard, three of my brightest

students, all in the same class, were diagnosed with MS," Moley told her. "One of them, a very brilliant young woman, became my assistant at *Newsweek*, and over the years I've watched her disease worsen. It's been heartbreaking."

As Moley spoke, his voice choked with emotion. He had witnessed just how devastating multiple sclerosis can be, and he had clearly been moved. At the end of the meeting, Sylvia asked him, "Would you consider joining our Board of Directors?" Without hesitation, he agreed.

Moley assumed the chairmanship of the Association's public education committee. He organized and presided over a press conference in New York City, designed to boost public visibility of the disease and the Society, and to educate the press, most of whom had never heard of MS. At that press conference, convened at the University Club in Manhattan, physicians such as Dr. Iago Galdston and Dr. Tracy Putnam described the nature of the disease and the ferocity with which it attacks the human body. They discussed theories about the causes of the disease, and the scarcity of treatments. Carl Owen talked about the organization's efforts to fund more research in the field.

Reporters also heard data from a study of hospital records in the Eastern Health District of Baltimore, which showed that in a ten-year period the number of people with MS who were admitted to hospitals was twice as high as the number hospitalized with polio. Sylvia's sister Alice, a research economist, had discovered this study while poring over the medical literature. It was a startling piece of statistical evidence indicating the scope of the MS problem. While people with polio were routinely hospitalized, most persons with MS were not, making the study's findings even more remarkable. Basil O'Connor, president of the National Foundation for Infantile Paralysis, called

Carl Owen when this statistic appeared in the press, complaining, "Carl, this is not fair play." He urged Owen to have the society stop using that statistic, particularly during the height of the fundraising campaign to support research for the polio vaccine. In deference to O'Connor, Owen agreed.

When Moley brought the press conference to a close, he commented, "The devil himself could not have contrived a more malevolent disease than multiple sclerosis."

The press conference produced a flurry of new attention for multiple sclerosis. Dozens of articles and editorials appeared. In the *New York Times*, Dr. Howard A. Rusk wrote that with the establishment of the Association for the Advancement of Research on Multiple Sclerosis, "the first wide-scale attack is being conducted on this ravaging and relatively common disease. The formation of the Association represents one of the most important steps that has been taken in this field."

For many readers, these articles were their first exposure to MS. They also offered hope to families who only recently had been confronted with the diagnosis of MS, and had not known where to turn.

Thacher Longstreth, who later became a Board member of the Society, recalled when his wife was diagnosed with multiple sclerosis. "In those days I didn't know anybody else who had MS," he said. "But here we were, with this disease affecting my wife, and when I asked the doctors where to go, they said, 'There's nowhere to go.' It was my first experience, except for some incidents in World War II, with how little doctors could do in some situations. I felt very frustrated. From that point up until this day, the one thing I want to see happen, more than anything else in the world, is the solution to multiple sclerosis."

Sylvia was determined that the Association would live up to its name and become a powerful force supporting research into MS. Research laboratories, she believed, would be the battlefields where the war against MS would be waged and eventually won. Her sister Alice wrote and produced a quarterly newsletter, *AARMS Forward,* with an initial mailing to two thousand people with MS and their family members to keep them abreast of developments in the research and treatment of multiple sclerosis and the organization's activities. Early solicitations for funds and membership dues emphasized that 100 percent of the contributions would be spent on research. Sylvia recalled, "Over the years, when I would ask people with MS and their families what they would like the Society to do for them, most would start by saying, 'Please find the answer.' In their minds, and in mine, that was the number one priority."

Other voluntary health organizations, such as the American Cancer Society, had never channeled all of their energy and money into research. But over the decades, Sylvia's early and continued emphasis on research has been widely praised, both inside and outside the society. Stephen Reingold, vice president of research programs at the National Multiple Sclerosis Society, says, "From the very beginning, Mrs. Lawry did something that was extraordinarily important in the evolution of our understanding of MS, and that was to stress research. She recognized that to solve the problems that were facing her brother and others with MS, science would need to be emphasized. She was not trained as a scientist herself; she was a concerned lay person. But she brought together medical advisers who helped her understand the world of science and the role of basic and clinical research. She also made it possible for other lay people to understand the importance of research."

"People knew that my motivation grew out of my brother's illness," Sylvia said. "But, in time, it became more than that. I got to know and care about so many people with MS and their families. So when money needed to be raised from individuals who didn't know much or anything about the disease, I could paint a very dramatic and realistic picture of the disease."

Sylvia didn't have to work hard to make the plight of people with MS seem poignant. Every day she received letters and phone calls from men and women with heartbreaking stories of ravaged lives. People described their anxiety upon experiencing their first symptoms. They told of their difficulty walking, or their panic as their vision became impaired. They spoke of tears and anger, depression and mourning, and painful acceptance of a relentless disease.

"By nature, I can't ask favors of people, let alone ask for money," said Sylvia. "But I found it easy to ask for funds for MS, because the need was so urgent, and the pain was so great."

8

THE MS RESEARCH MISSION could be led only by experts—a Medical Advisory Board which in turn could recognize and reward viable research projects. The Association's board consisted of some of the best minds in the field of neurology. Dr. H. Houston Merritt, a pioneer neurologist, had developed the anti-epilepsy drug Dilantin with Dr. Tracy Putnam. Dr. Merritt had conducted basic scientific research into many central nervous system diseases and had devised techniques for accurately measuring the cerebrospinal fluid surrounding the brain and spinal cord, associating fluid abnormalities with various diseases. In the Association's earliest days, he was chief neurologist at Montefiore Hospital in the Bronx, and in 1948 he became chairman of Columbia University's neurology department and director of the Neurological Institute in New York.

Dr. Merritt sat through Medical Advisory Board meetings barely uttering a word until near the end, when he would offer his observations and conclusions in a few words, almost instantly resolving the issue at hand. One of his fellow neurologists described Dr. Merritt this way: "His deductive-reasoning senses work a mile a minute and his mind works so fast that one sometimes has difficulty following how he arrives at his astute conclusions."

Dr. Thomas Rivers, director of the Rockefeller Institute and its affiliated hospital, was the first vice chairman of the Medical Advisory Board. He was widely recognized as an authority on viral diseases, and his contributions to the study of polio had played a role in the development of the Salk and Sabin vaccines. While still in medical school, Dr. Rivers had been diagnosed with a serious illness called progressive central muscular atrophy of the Aran-Duchenne type, and although he was given just months to live, he exceeded those expectations by many decades. Though strong-willed, opinionated, and outspoken, he often referred to himself as just a country boy from Georgia. He strongly believed that the answers to many devastating diseases, including MS, lay in careful, methodical laboratory research.

In 1926, Dr. Rivers had conducted studies in which he repeatedly injected brain tissue from one monkey into another, which in the recipient animal produced a paralytic, demyelinating condition comparable to MS. It was a breakthrough that had laid the groundwork for many studies that would follow, and it made Rivers a logical choice for membership on the Medical Advisory Board.

With Drs. Putnam, Merritt, and Rivers as guides, the Association began awarding its first research grants. An anonymous donation of more than $54,000 funded the very first grant. Although the donor insisted on anonymity at the time, he had signed the check, thereby divulging his identity as a prominent New York lawyer and financier. Sylvia never learned why the donor had an interest in supporting MS research, but he had earmarked the money for the research of Dr. Elvin Kabat, a brilliant young scientist at Columbia University College of Physicians and Surgeons. In June 1947 the Association formally awarded Kabat those funds for a three-year study investigating the ways in which the immune system affected the brain and spinal cord in multiple sclerosis, and the role that allergic responses might play in MS.

Dr. Tracy Putnam couldn't contain his enthusiasm. "Here we are, in our first year, and we're already making our first research grant," he said. "It usually takes an organization like this about five years to get a research program off the ground." Another investigator believed that Dr. Kabat's research might have implications beyond MS, describing the study as an "important step toward combating a major crippling disease. It also may well be that this research will throw light on other kindred nervous disorders."

Dr. Kabat's research team worked with an animal model that closely resembled MS. Like Dr. Rivers before them, Dr. Kabat and his colleagues used normal monkeys in which they stimulated brain injury through injections of brain tissue. The animals developed a paralytic condition similar to MS, even to the point of having remissions. When Carl Owen and Sylvia Lawry visited Dr. Kabat's lab, he showed them just how close the animal model was to MS in humans, inserting a stick through the cage bars directly in the line of sight of a monkey; but the animal could not see the stick because of its MS-like visual impairment.

By 1948, in his studies of human spinal fluid, Dr. Kabat had found abnormalities in the immunological proteins in people with MS. Laboratory evaluations showed that these proteins formed unique patterns called oligoclonal bands. Dr. Kabat's findings not only demonstrated a direct link between

MS and the immune system but also suggested that the detection of these bands might be used to help diagnose the disease.

In the months that followed, the Society funded a steady stream of studies. Dr. Albert Harris of Albany General Hospital received a grant to study the spinal fluid of persons with MS, searching for unique factors in the fluid that might be different from those individuals without the disease. Dr. Gabriel Steiner, a neurologist at Wayne State and a member of the Medical Advisory Board, was awarded funds for a three-year study of the theory that an infectious agent caused MS.

As the Association's research program progressed, Carl Owen immersed himself in the medical literature about multiple sclerosis and sat in at every Medical Advisory Board meeting. He asked pointed questions and quickly earned the respect of the physicians. At one meeting Owen asked, "Why don't you doctors approach a problem like multiple sclerosis the way we lawyers approach a problem? Why don't you assemble all the known facts about MS, try to define what the gaps in knowledge are, and proceed to recruit people to fill those gaps?" Dr. Rivers responded, "We don't yet know enough about the nervous system in healthy people to focus on MS in that way."

The Medical Advisory Board believed that basic scientific research would provide clues to areas that seemed most promising for MS. Thus the board recommended grants in areas ranging from virology to immunology to genetics. Investigators began studying the essential structure and function of living tissues and their metabolism, in both healthy and diseased states. They probed for information on how tissues reacted to chemical and physical stimuli. They also conducted clinical research concerned with the entire human structure, not just particular tissues and organs, evaluating the body's response to specific medical and physical therapies.

At the same time the Association sponsored a statistical survey to determine the incidence of MS in New York City and the surrounding region. In 1947, guided by Dr. John Zabriskie of the Neurological Institute, questionnaires were mailed to all the physicians (more than seventeen thousand) in the metropolitan New York area, including parts of New Jersey and Connecticut, requesting the number of persons with MS under their care, as well as the names of these people to avoid duplication among those being treated by more than one doctor. About 10 percent of the physicians completed and returned the questionnaire. Survey data were compiled by Sylvia's two sisters, Alice and Lillian, along with Lillian's best friend. Even with the survey's limited sample size, more than five thousand cases of MS were reported in the New York area. "Our Medical Advisory Board thought this was a remarkably high number," said Sylvia. "At the time, many physicians weren't familiar enough with MS symptoms to make an accurate diagnosis. So there were certainly many undiagnosed cases that we never heard about, plus thousands of other people with MS being cared for by doctors who did not respond to the survey."

The research program created enormous hopes among Association members. "When I attended meetings with the people involved in trying to conquer MS, there was a real sense that we could do it in a few years," said lay board member L. Palmer Brown. "I felt that a ten-year time frame was safe, although others believed that we'd have answers in five years. I became very committed to help raise money that was needed for research, and getting this terrible disease behind us. With my wife in the early stages of MS at the time, this was especially important to me."

Chapter 8

With the hope that a cure was in sight, the Association accelerated its efforts to raise money. In 1947, Carl Owen approached a nationally prominent fundraising organization, the same firm that had coordinated campaigns for the American Cancer Society. Owen asked for its participation in raising $100,000, and felt confident that the organization would come on board. But a few days later he received a letter from one of the firm's executives, declining Owen's request. He told Owen, "We couldn't raise $100,000 for you. Multiple sclerosis is not like cancer or heart disease; most of the public has never heard of MS, and knows nothing about it. To make the task even more difficult, you don't have sufficient volunteers in place to benefit from our guidance. To raise that kind of money, you need more volunteers."

Owen was incensed by the rejection. "I'm going to raise the $100,000 myself!" he told Sylvia. "Every penny of it!" And he did. In the upcoming weeks, Owen asked nearly everyone he encountered for contributions. Once he had explained the effects of MS on the lives of families, no one said "no," often out of friendship and respect for Owen. Some of the donations were modest; others were much more significant. Before the end of the year he had reached the $100,000 goal, and had done it single-handedly.

9

As SYLVIA READ and responded to the mountain of letters that came into the office each day, one fact became undeniable: people with MS had immediate needs that could not wait to be addressed. Some required home care, physical therapy, or rehabilitation. Others, given their physical limitations, needed help in obtaining employment. Many required the services of social workers, therapists, and other counselors. Almost all of them needed information, from answers to their most basic question—"What is MS?"—to referrals to medical centers and other service providers.

As important as research was to Sylvia and to the Board of Directors, these daily needs of people with multiple sclerosis cried out to be met. With few exceptions, no one was providing any help. "Many people with MS felt that their plight was overwhelming, and that their need for services was so great," Sylvia observed. The answer, she decided, was community-based chapters that could provide services and education, and conduct fundraising on their own.

"Of course, it was important never to lose sight of research, so I continued to hammer away at how crucial it was," Sylvia said. "It was still of paramount importance. The board also decided that in every way possible we would seize opportunities to design programs to help people live with their illness. And chapters seemed like a good way to do that."

In July 1947 the mission of the Association expanded beyond research. It also changed its name. It officially became known as the National Multiple Sclerosis Society.

The first chapters were launched in California and Connecticut. Board member Henry J. Kaiser, Jr., was the driving force behind the California chapter. Kaiser had been diagnosed with MS in 1944 while overseeing the Kaiser-operated artillery shell plants in Colorado and California. He was zealous in his efforts to fight the disease. The Connecticut chapter was started by Georgina Davids, an indefatigable woman with MS who used a wheelchair. She had been commissioner of welfare for the State of Connecticut, and had a sophisticated knowledge of how an organization should be run. Davids solicited the support of Nancy Carnegie Rockefeller, wife of the banker James Stillman Rockefeller, who helped get the Connecticut group off the ground.

The early chapters had limited financial and manpower resources. But they took the critical first steps toward launching programs at the local level to help people with MS and to direct them to service providers in the community. They became an invaluable source of information for families coping with the disease. They made referrals to physicians and other health-care professionals who had some expertise in MS. They helped find resources for caring for house-bound individuals. They organized meetings in which people with MS could meet others with the disease and attend lectures by local physicians who answered many questions. The chapters also made their first attempts at fundraising.

From the beginning, the MS Society instituted a policy used by the American Cancer Society—spending 60 percent of the funds raised by the chapters on local programs while delivering 40 percent to the national organization for research projects approved by the Medical Advisory Board. It sounded like a workable system, at least on paper. The chapters, however, were just learning to fundraise, and there was no professional input to guide them in that effort. At times they struggled in their campaigns to raise money, and they debated where to spend their limited resources. As the number of chapters eventually increased, the financial pressures seemed only to grow, particularly as local demands increased.

One chapter chairperson explained it bluntly to Sylvia: "If I visit an MS patient and find him sprawled on the floor and not able to get himself back in bed, I'm not going to worry about research! My first concern is providing the services he needs."

In what seemed like no time at all, the number of Society chapters mushroomed. Board member Paul Voorhies, a Detroit attorney and president of the Kresge Foundation, founded a chapter in Michigan. Voorhies had a son with MS. In rapid succession, chapters were formed in Alabama, Minnesota, Massachusetts, Vermont, Eastern Pennsylvania, Kings County and Nassau County, New York, and Racine, Wisconsin. Besides providing crucial information and coordinating essential services in their areas, these chapters also pushed to stimulate interest in MS among medical researchers in their communities.

Local leadership was often assumed by people who had written to the national office expressing an interest in starting a chapter. More often than not, these individuals were given approval. Their management skills varied, however. Some chapters lagged far behind others in organizing communities and reaching out to local researchers.

Nevertheless the existence of the local chapters helped meet one of the Society's greatest challenges, and one that was altogether intangible. Individuals with multiple sclerosis often found their lives crushed, and they withdrew from the remaining joys of living. Through the hands-on work of the local chapters, the Society was able to help individuals with MS renew their self-confidence and instill in them a belief that they could have a future.

Even as the chapters formed one after another and the outreach of the Society grew, the national office continued to operate on a shoestring. Sylvia monitored every penny that came across her desk. Somehow the phone and electricity bills got paid, and money was found for stamps and envelopes. The lack of funds, however, was a constant source of pressure. At times there was a climate of near hysteria in the organization. Yet the work went on. When a researcher submitted a grant application for a worthwhile project, the board searched for sources to fund it. When Sylvia's workload became overwhelming, she and the board finally decided to hire a secretary. Her name was Sally Whitcup, and she came on only part-time. Even so, part-time often stretched into the evening hours. "There was so much work to do, and she desperately needed help," said Sally. "We'd barely stop for meals. We might have sandwiches sent up, gobble them down in fifteen minutes, and then get back to work."

Sally was married to Leonard Whitcup, a well-known songwriter and vice president of the Songwriters Guild. He had written the popular tunes "Take Me Back to My Boots and Saddle,"

"From the Vine Came the Grape," and "Bewildered." Leonard often came to the office in the evening and insisted that his wife wrap up her work for the night. Otherwise Sally might have remained at her desk for many more hours.

Carl Owen did the same thing. He often stopped by at seven or eight at night after leaving his law office. He had to convince Sylvia to grab a cup of coffee with him. "There will always be work," he told her. "You need a break for a few minutes."

Meanwhile Sylvia's marriage had ended in divorce. She was convinced that her brother's illness did not contribute to the breakup. After the divorce, she continued to work at the Society. Her sister Alice generously gave Sylvia half her salary, allowing Sylvia to work at the Society without drawing a paycheck. The goal of the family was to help Bernard, and they were all willing to sacrifice to do so.

"Bernie kept me focused on the Society," Sylvia said. "Everything of significance related to MS was coming into the office, and as I gave each bit of news to him, it made him more optimistic."

It was optimism that often eluded Sylvia as she struggled to keep the Society afloat. "The need for services was so great, and the resources were so limited," Sylvia said. "None of us knew what the next day would bring. But there was always the hope that the next day would provide the answer to multiple sclerosis."

10

IN 1948 an editorial in the *New York Times* carried the head-line "A Challenge to Medicine." It praised the National MS Society for what it had already achieved but stressed that only a start had been made. "Thousands of patients are pleading for treatment and training opportunities," the editorial stated. "Basic research projects are awaiting investigation, and technical training of personnel in the methodology of the management of the problem is sorely needed." The editorial concluded with words that Sylvia Lawry already knew. "There is no more challenging problem facing medicine today than multiple sclerosis."

Despite the enormity of the task, Sylvia had cause for optimism. In September 1948 a three-year, $50,000 grant from the Milbank Memorial Fund allowed the Society to appoint its first medical director. Dr. Cornelius H. Traeger was an influential rheumatologist in New York City with a successful Park Avenue practice. His patients included Robert Sarnoff, John Gunther, and Mary Lasker. But Dr. Traeger was seeking new interests and challenges. He found them in MS.

Until Dr. Traeger's arrival, Sylvia had been responding to medical questions from the public as best she could, often making calls to Medical Advisory Board members for factual information. Dr. Traeger relieved her of some of those responsibilities and directed the medical arm of the organization. During his tenure as medical director, he helped organize medical advisory committees at the local level. He was convinced of the urgency of conducting MS research, and when he felt that a particular research project needed to be done but no funds were available for it, he would go out and raise them.

Although Dr. Traeger brought needed expertise to the day-to-day operations of the Society, he insisted that Sylvia still attend meetings dealing with the medical aspects of the disease. He knew that she had read most of the scientific literature on MS, and he often called upon her own expertise. "Dr. Traeger and I worked very well together," Sylvia recalled. "At the time I was in my mid-thirties and he was in his mid-fifties. But even within his own circle this highly respected doctor would introduce me as his boss."

Dr. Traeger had the uncanny ability to discuss multiple sclerosis in ways that the general public could understand and that could persuade prominent people to lend their influence to the MS movement. He oversaw educational efforts for both laymen and physicians, and recruited Cornell University neurologist George A. Schumacher to write a comprehensive manual on MS, covering its cause, diagnosis, treatment, and rehabilitation. That manual became the medical bible on multiple sclerosis for years. It was mailed to 76,000 physicians throughout the country and was printed in the *Journal of the American Medical Association.*

Dr. Schumacher, who later became chairman of the National Society's Medical Advisory Board, concluded his expansive report this way: "No case of unequivocal cure of established multiple sclerosis is on record. No case of complete relief of symptoms of significant duration has been proved to be due to a therapeutic measure." Then he added, "The outlook for cure of the disease by use of drugs is unpromising." Nevertheless, by the early 1950s Schumacher was predicting that the answer to MS would be found within five years.

In 1948 the first MS clinics became part of the National Society's clinical research program. They were created at Boston State Hospital, Albany (New York) Hospital, New York University–Bellevue Medical Center, and Snyder Jones Clinic in Winfield, Kansas. Chapter-affiliated clinics that concentrated on services were established at facilities such as Massachusetts General Hospital in Boston, Los Angeles' Cedars of Lebanon Hospital, Stanford University Hospital, Rhode Island Hospital in Providence, St. Luke's Hospital in Chicago, and Yale University Medical Center in New Haven. People with MS often turned to the clinics for evaluations, diagnosis, treatment, and physical therapy at nominal fees. At the same time these clinics became important for MS researchers. As a National Multiple Sclerosis Society statement declared, "It is through such clinics that the progress of disease symptoms can be charted and therapy effectiveness can be evaluated best."

During the final days of 1948, the National MS Society announced its plans to raise $225,000 to support an all-out assault on MS. At a press conference to launch the fundraising effort, Arthur Clark, a man with MS, described the compelling need for meaningful research, and how the disease had turned his own life upside down. "You walk down the street of your hometown, and people think you're drunk," he said. "Maybe they say you've got polio. But there isn't one in a thousand who knows that you've really got multiple sclerosis."

Although the National Multiple Sclerosis Society continued to support several clinics across the country, individuals
with MS desperately sought help wherever they could find it.
Sometimes they were drawn to worthless therapies that drained
them of both optimism and money. The treatments initially
promised a glimmer of hope but in the end only crushed their
spirits. Sylvia's brother Bernard tried one of these therapies. It
was being promoted by Henry J. Kaiser, Jr., a National Society
board member and founder of the California chapter.

At the age of twenty-seven, Kaiser had been diagnosed with
MS. Three years later he joined the board at the urging of his
father, head of the Kaiser steel dynasty. The elder Kaiser was a
client of Carl Owen's, and when Owen approached him to
serve on the board, Kaiser recommended his son instead. He
was the first person with MS to enter the Society's leadership
ranks.

Before long, Henry Kaiser, Jr., became an outspoken proponent of rigorous physical therapy as a primary treatment for
multiple sclerosis. In conjunction with a physiatrist, he established the Kabat-Kaiser Institutes for Physical Medicine in MS,
which offered the hope of a cure through aggressive physical
therapy and rehabilitation. Theirs was a radically different approach from the sedentary lifestyle recommended at the time
by most doctors. For people who been inactive for years, the
Kabat-Kaiser approach presented something of a physical
shock, but Kaiser believed that he was being cured by the program. "He tried to convince the Society to get behind the program and raise money for the Institutes," said Sylvia. When
Reader's Digest published an article by Paul de Kruif that was
highly complimentary of the Kabat-Kaiser Institutes and their
treatment of MS, Kaiser turned up the pressure on the Society
to help establish and fund more Kabat-Kaiser sites and make re-

ferrals to them. "Our Medical Advisory Board was very skeptical," said Sylvia. "So was our Board of Directors. No one thought that physical therapy would be the ultimate answer."

With the *Reader's Digest*–generated wave of interest in the Kabat-Kaiser Institutes, Bernard expressed interest in trying the new therapy. With some apprehension, Sylvia sent her brother to California to undergo six months of muscular "re-education"—and to test whether Kaiser was right. Bernard began the strenuous exercise and physiotherapy program. Like others, he was encouraged to move his arms and legs against light resistance that was gradually increased as his muscles became stronger. He pushed himself to the limit—and beyond.

As a result, Bernard's hopes for deliverance from MS were shattered in California. "As it turned out, he had an absolutely disastrous experience there," Sylvia remembered. Bernard did regain some mobility, and before long he was able to walk farther and with less of a stagger than before his arrival. He worked very hard on parallel bars and, desperate to get better, drove himself to physical and emotional exhaustion.

"The basic concept of the Kabat-Kaiser program was to perform passive resistance exercises to the point of fatigue—an approach that is no longer recommended," Sylvia said. "Bernie was like me; whatever he did, he had to do it well. So he would work on the parallel bars alone until the wee hours of the night. But he overdid it. One night I got a call that he had suffered an emotional collapse. I flew out to the West Coast to bring him home. He had suffered a nervous breakdown and an exacerbation of the MS. All the benefits he had achieved at Kabat-Kaiser were soon gone."

When the National Society refused to yield to Henry Kaiser, Jr.'s request for support, he resigned from the board and relinquished his chairmanship of the California chapter.

Although the Kabat-Kaiser Institutes continued to operate, they put much less emphasis on MS.

After Bernard's visit to the Kabat-Kaiser Institutes, he was treated by Molly Harrower, a clinical psychologist and member of the Medical Advisory Board. Harrower made an important contribution to the movement by promoting support groups for persons with MS after observing the first such group in action in Connecticut. With a Society grant, Harrower also wrote manuals on the mental health of MS patients, which provided guidance to neurologists, psychologists, and other health-care professionals. Harrower was able to guide Bernard out of his psychological distress. Her contribution was significant in the struggle against a disease that struck on so many levels.

11

SYLVIA LAWRY knew that the success of the Society she had founded depended on greater public awareness of multiple sclerosis. The disease had to be recognizable to every American. The media were crucial to this effort. Effectively reaching them was a skill that Sylvia dearly wanted to perfect.

One of the masters in the field of publicity was Edward Bernays, a man the *New York Times* called "the father of public relations." A nephew of Sigmund Freud, Bernays considered himself a professional opinion maker, a person who could change public attitudes. It was an art he had been practicing since the 1920s. Bernays's client list included General Electric, Procter & Gamble, General Motors, CBS, NBC, and Time Inc. When Procter & Gamble became concerned that children were complaining that soap was stinging their eyes, Bernays created a national soap sculpture contest that ultimately involved 22 million kids and had them associating soap with fun rather than eye irritation. He handled publicity for Samuel Goldwyn and Clare Booth Luce. He counseled Herbert Hoover, Henry Ford, and Thomas Edison. In the late 1940s he advised the government of India on how to promote democracy. To transform Calvin Coolidge's sullen public image, Bernays invited Al Jolson and an array of starlets to the White House for breakfast, then issued a press release claiming that Coolidge had been the life of the party.

When Sylvia learned that Otto Frohnknecht, one of the Society's early supporters, was a relative of Bernays, she asked Frohnknecht to arrange a "top-level cultivation." She knew of Bernays's involvement with a contest supporting research into cancer and heart disease on the popular program "Truth or Consequences," which was sponsored by Procter & Gamble. To win prizes, the public submitted entries that completed the statement, "I should support heart research because . . ." The contest helped raised more than $1 million and was the basis upon which the American Heart Association became a national organization. Why couldn't the same be done for MS?

Accompanied by a leading neurologist, Sylvia met with Bernays at the University Club in New York and pled the case for his involvement in gaining public support for multiple sclerosis. Lawry painted a poignant picture of people with the disease, how it devastated their lives and those of their families. She spoke of the desperate need for research and treatment, and suggested that an effort like the "Truth or Consequences" campaign could do wonders.

Bernays listened politely. Then he told Sylvia, "Well, that was a very fine performance!" Then, after giving it a few moments of thought, he said, "As much as I'd like to do this for you, it wouldn't be in the interest of Procter & Gamble. The words 'multiple sclerosis' are entirely new to me, and I'm sure that's the case with most people. Our audience won't know what multiple sclerosis is or why they should support it. A lot of them won't even be able to say or spell it. I think if we featured multiple sclerosis on our show, it would narrow audience participation in our contest, and that would not be acceptable to my client."

Sylvia was shattered. Yet the meeting turned out to be a crucial step in the young history of the MS movement. Bernays was intrigued by Sylvia's enthusiasm and dedication, and at her request he agreed to become a member of the Society's National Board in 1949. He also was appointed chairman of the Society's Public Relations Advisory Committee, succeeding Raymond Moley, the former presidential adviser.

Bernays confessed that he was quite taken with Lawry during that first meeting. "She was a very charming young woman, and she started talking about her brother who was sick with a disease I had never heard of, and said she was so moved by his plight that she had started a Society," he said. "It seemed that she had devoted her entire life to helping her brother and people like him. Without any previous experience in the field, without money, and with the disadvantage of being a woman in a man's world—she was determined to do something constructive and concrete. She made quite an impression on me."

According to Bernays, his meeting with Sylvia occurred in an era when women were not taken seriously enough. That made Sylvia Lawry's accomplishments all the more astonishing. "My wife was my partner for fifty-eight years, but I never used her name on our letterhead because clients would have thought she was interested only in fashion, lipstick, or food," said Bernays. "If I had taken her to meetings at General Motors, they wouldn't have listened to anything she said. Those were the circumstances that women faced. Sylvia was trying to get things done at a time when women were simply brushed aside.

It would be like a woman wanting to run for president of the United States in 1910. People would have just shrugged their shoulders. I'm sure Sylvia encountered attitudes like that."

Said Sylvia, "Eddie Bernays was extraordinary. He became my mentor and taught me a good deal about the dynamics of PR." As Sylvia recruited people for fundraising leadership roles and for National Board membership, Bernays advised her, "Keep your eye on page one of the *New York Times*; the people who make page one are those you should go after." When she'd present him with a list of possible candidates, he'd focus her attention on their influence in the community—the corporate boards they sat on, their social connections, and the leverage they might bring to the National MS Society. They analyzed the candidates one by one, determining the comparative value. Then, relying on chutzpah and her skills at persuasion, Sylvia went directly into the nation's largest corporate offices—sometimes with the help of impressive letters of introduction—asking CEOs and presidents for help.

Bernays also suggested that the Society emphasize the term "MS" rather than "multiple sclerosis." He said, "It will be easier for people to remember two letters of the alphabet rather than long words that they can't say and can't spell. By calling it 'multiple sclerosis,' it's like asking the public to accept a Latin or Greek term as if it were a breakfast cereal like shredded wheat."

For the next four decades Bernays made MS one of his crusades. He masterfully made the disease recognizable to millions of Americans. To Sylvia, his guidance was invaluable. "In my everyday activities, from the day I met him, I was guided by what Edward Bernays would have had me do," she said.

When Bernays was one hundred years old, Sylvia spent a day with him at his home in Cambridge, Massachusetts. He was as spry and vital as ever. He told her he was writing a book "about my second hundred years." He said he had taken a test which showed that while his chronological age was one hundred, he was functioning physically and mentally as though he were sixty-three. He spent much of their time together trying to persuade her to write a book about her life fighting MS. "You owe it to the women's lib movement," he said.

Bernays died three years later at age 103.

12

THE CORE MISSION of the Society continued to be research, something Sylvia Lawry believed was the only hope for her brother Bernard and all MS patients. The Society was true to its goal of devoting as much of its funds as possible to this research. A survey conducted by the Albert and Mary Lasker Foundation in 1951, which determined how the nation's nine leading voluntary health agencies spent their money, ranked the MS Society as the leader in the proportion of funds channeled into research. In 1948, 1949, and 1950, the Society spent 42 percent, 64 percent, and 42 percent, respectively, of its income on research. That was far greater than the second-ranked agency, which appropriated an average 25 percent of its funds for research.

In those early years the Society had no specific research agenda. Because little was still known about the nervous systems of healthy people, let alone those with multiple sclerosis, members of the Medical Advisory Board acknowledged that, in a sense, they were on a fishing expedition. Gradually the Society's research efforts achieved a maturity and direction, supporting quality research in all areas that might solve the mysteries surrounding the disease. Scientists approached the organization with applications for MS research in their own fields of interest. The Society's Medical Advisory Board reviewed the applications and submitted its recommendations to the lay Board of Directors, which made the final funding decisions.

The Medical Advisory Board recognized that progress against MS would depend on the efforts of both laboratory scientists and clinical investigators, and a coordination of their efforts. Some grants supported basic research, investigating the fundamental structure of tissues and organs. Others funded clinical research, evaluating the disease process of MS, its symptomatology, and patient responses to drug treatments and physical therapy.

At the Neurological Institute in New York City, researchers examined the effects of a pituitary gland secretion, ACTH (adrenocorticotropic hormone), on the course of MS. At the Southwest Institute of Applied Research in Texas, scientists looked for evidence of a possible viral origin of MS. At Boston State Hospital, clinicians probed the patterns and possible explanations for spontaneous remissions in people with MS. At the Massachusetts General Hospital and the Harvard Medical School, investigators explored the basic nature of myelin and the process of myelin degradation—demyelination.

At the urging of the Society, the Association for Research in Nervous and Mental Diseases devoted its entire December 1948 conference to MS. More than thirty scientific papers were presented at the conference, providing an overview of what was already known about MS, the theories of what caused and might treat the disease, and the challenges ahead. This comprehensive analysis by many of the nation's leading neurologists gave the Society a strong foundation for raising funds to support specific research projects in a variety of areas.

As Sylvia sought new sources of research support, she turned her attention to the federal government. To her dismay, she discovered that up to 1949 the National Institutes of Health had made only one grant for MS research. The total amount: $14,000. At the time, all government-sponsored neurological research was funded through the National Institute of Mental Health, whose governing committees were composed largely of psychiatrists, not neurologists. So when research funds were being appropriated, MS received almost nothing.

Nonetheless Sylvia recognized that the government's potential for research support was enormous and could dwarf the Society's own fundraising success. The Society shouldn't be alone in financing research, she said. On several occasions she told Dr. Traeger, "If we're going to win this war, we absolutely have to get the government involved." All that remained was a plan to convince lawmakers in Washington that the battle against MS was worth fighting.

Then, quite unexpectedly, Sylvia received a phone call from U.S. Senator Charles Tobey of New Hampshire, whose daughter had been diagnosed with multiple sclerosis. "What can I do to help?" he asked her. And then he added, "What do you think of me introducing a bill to form an MS Institute to support research?"

It was just what Sylvia wanted to hear. A government-sponsored MS Institute, under the umbrella of the National Institutes of Health, could become a steady source of research dollars. Senator Tobey agreed to lead the charge within the halls of Congress, and eventually fourteen bills were introduced to establish the new institute. Most congressmen had never heard of MS and asked their colleagues what it was all about.

As part of the campaign for an MS Institute, Dr. Traeger began negotiating with Dr. Leonard Sheely, the U.S. surgeon general. Dr. Sheely stubbornly resisted the concept of establishing an institute devoted solely to MS. "There are more than four hundred neurological diseases," he told Dr. Traeger (in the year 2000 there were more than six hundred), "and it simply doesn't make sense to create a separate MS Institute. Other groups will press us for institutes for their particular diseases, and it could get completely out of hand. It's a bad idea."

Rather than giving up, the National MS Society offered a compromise—the establishment of a National Institute for Neurological Diseases and Blindness that would fund all neurological conditions, including MS (its name was later changed to the National Institute for Neurological Disorders and Stroke, or NINDS). Dr. Traeger pointed out to the surgeon general that persons with an interest in nearly every other neurological disease had often approached the National MS Society, asking the Society for funds that they could use for their own programs and research. "You've got to develop a 'citizens' budget' that will take care of the needs of all of these people," he told the government representatives.

Senator Tobey held his ground, lobbying for an MS Institute in order to attract public attention to multiple sclerosis, with the compromise proposal of a broader-based institute to be considered at a later date. Before long, however, it seemed time to shift energies toward supporting a more encompassing Neurological Diseases Institute. Sylvia coordinated an aggressive campaign in support of it. Chapter members wrote thousands of letters and made thousands of phone calls to their congressmen. Neurologists lobbied in the Capitol. New York philanthropist Mary Lasker, who played a major role in the success of the American Cancer Society, lent her support to the MS Society's campaign, and at her suggestion Sylvia maintained a lobbyist, Norman Winter, to push the cause forward.

To ensure that multiple sclerosis would receive the attention it deserved in the new agency, Sylvia organized a group of MS experts to travel to Washington in May 1949 to testify before the Senate Labor and Public Welfare Subcommittee that was considering establishment of the institute. The society's team was headed by Drs. Tracy Putnam and H. Houston Merritt, chairman and vice chairman, respectively, of the Medical Advisory Board. (As usual, Sylvia monitored every dollar that was spent on that Washington trip, even arranging for the two physicians to share a hotel room. But she had been unaware of a strained relationship between the men; they weren't even on speaking terms.) Their testimony focused on the crisis of multiple sclerosis and the pressing need to find answers for the disease. "My hope was not only to create momentum for the creation of the Institute, but also to increase public awareness of MS," said Sylvia.

The public and the press packed the hearing room. Spectators included many people with MS, some in wheelchairs. Senator Tobey opened the hearings by calling MS "this hellish disease." Dr. Traeger testified, "Some people have ventured the thought that perhaps MS is an increasing disease because it has something to do with the strain of living in our modern civilization. If that is true, we are facing a dangerous situation in this country."

The star witness was Eleanor Gehrig, the widow of the famed New York Yankee first baseman who had been forced to retire because of amyotrophic lateral sclerosis, a motor neuron disease which, like MS, is a demyelinating disease. Earlier that year the Society had established the Lou Gehrig Memorial Fund, which served as an effective vehicle for educating Americans about the goals and accomplishments of the organization. The fund was created as a living tribute to Gehrig, who died in 1941, two years after leaving baseball.

Sylvia had convinced Gehrig's widow of the need to testify at the congressional hearings. "We needed someone who would capture the public's imagination, and around whom we could build some publicity," recalled Sylvia. "Mrs. Gehrig was able to create immediate public recognition of the kind of problem MS is." Although Sylvia, Society board members, and a number of physicians also testified, Mrs. Gehrig's words were the most dramatic. She told a spellbound panel of senators how her husband's illness had undermined his baseball career and shattered his life. She described the importance of research to reduce human suffering. Her testimony made headlines across the country, including a *New York Times* article that carried the banner, "Mrs. Gehrig Backs Sclerosis Aid Bill."

In August 1950, Congress voted to create the new Neurological Institute. President Harry Truman signed the bill into law.

The establishment of the National Institute for Neurological Diseases and Blindness, with Dr. Pearce Bailey as its first director, represented a milestone in the war against multiple sclerosis. Government appropriations for neurological diseases, including MS, escalated dramatically almost overnight. The first government appropriation was $1.2 million in 1952, divided among all the neurological diseases, including MS; the following year funding increased to $4.5 million, and to $7.7 million in 1954. As available funds for research and training programs soared, many more scientists became interested in conducting MS studies. Dr. Merritt called the establishment of the Institute the greatest single factor in raising the level of neurological research and increasing interest in neurology as a medical specialty in the United States. At the same time Dr. Traeger and Sylvia Lawry formed the National Committee for Research in Neurological Diseases—a coalition of leaders representing all the neurological conditions. It became a lobbying instrument in Washington, speaking in one voice and designed to ensure that each neurological condition was being fairly funded through the new Institute.

From the beginning, the National MS Society had an excellent relationship with the Institute, sharing their respective data and coordinating their funding efforts. The federal agency was expected to fund broad basic neurologic research, leaving the National MS Society to concentrate on MS-targeted research. Since the 1950s the government and the Society have supported virtually every major multiple sclerosis study in the United States. The creation of the Institute, and its positive and productive working relationship with the Society, strengthened Sylvia's hopes that the answers for MS were imminent.

13

No one was more important to Sylvia Lawry and the MS Society in its formative years than Carl Owen, the Society's first president. So when he suffered a serious heart attack, it hit Sylvia hard. Owen eventually died of heart disease in 1954 at his winter residence in Delray Beach, Florida, at the age of seventy-four. Before his death, Owen handpicked his successor, New York businessman and philanthropist Ralph I. Straus.

When Straus assumed the presidency, Sylvia was confronted with a stunning turn of events. Straus was intent on stimulating the growth of the Society—a goal that had unanimous support. Toward that end, he sat down with Sylvia and asked her to step aside. He told her that she did not have the background necessary to be the Society's top executive. "I hear that you're doing a wonderful job, Sylvia," he told her. "But I doubt that a woman, particularly a young woman like you, will be able to attract top-level professional men to serve under you."

Sylvia was stunned. Carl Owen had always shown complete confidence in her. When Owen met people who contemplated making a contribution to the Society, he told them, "I'd like you to meet Sylvia Lawry and have her tell you something about MS." She convinced them of the importance and the urgency of conquering the disease. "I could paint a dramatic picture of the disease; people could see that my motivation came out of my brother's illness and my concern for the many persons with MS and their families whom I've met," she said.

When Sylvia prepared reports for the Society that needed Owen's attention, he told her, "These reports are as good as any that I've received from the attorneys at my law office." He sometimes said that as executive head of the Society, she was doing all the work and he was just riding her coattails. He joked, "The only leadership qualities you're lacking are that you're not fat and grey!" And he added, "But gold is where you find it."

Straus, however, was concerned about Sylvia's status in the Society. In his mind, she didn't fit the male stereotype of someone capable of running a fast-growing organization. "It came as a surprise that Ralph Straus would make a judgment without having really worked with me," she said. "So I was shocked out of concern for the future of the Society, although I put up no resistance at all." She acquiesced immediately, saying she would cooperate in any way to promote the Society's goals.

In terms of titles and appearances, the National Society's hierarchy changed. Sylvia no longer held the title of the organization's chief executive but was asked by Straus to continue on as executive secretary. Her work never stopped. "I didn't start the Society with the dream of becoming an executive," she said. "I never felt I had a lien on the job. But because I was doing all the work, it just followed that I would take on the title because there wasn't enough money to pay a high salary. Carl

Owen had confidence in me, which gave me the confidence that I could do it. So I did."

Sylvia's mission remained unchanged—to help fund research that would find a cure for multiple sclerosis. She didn't need an impressive title to keep her eyes focused on that prize. It wouldn't be long, however, until Straus's decision proved to be disastrous.

Before then, in 1951, the National MS Society issued its first annual report, which Straus described as a document intended "to convey a record of the results of five years of effort by the workers and contributors of the Society in its search for the cause and control of the complex disease symptoms called multiple sclerosis." In the report he noted that the Society had grown to a membership of more than nineteen thousand and had spent $324,632 on research grants to date.

But he cautioned that the bulk of the Society's funds were coming "from a relatively few individuals," and in order to carry on the organization's work "we need to enlist the support of many new friends. The needs are great and even with the most careful handling, our funds are inadequate." At that time about 70 percent of the Society's financial support was coming from members, their families, and other small contributors. The remainder was raised from charitable foundations. While the Society pointed with pride to the active interest of its members in offering support, despite their limited resources in many cases, it needed to broaden its base of support.

At the local level, the number of chapters was steadily increasing. By August 1951 there were sixteen chapters, which had collectively transmitted nearly $80,000 to the national office since their formation. Chapters formed their own medical programs, guided by local medical advisory boards. They attempted to stimulate medical interest and research in MS, and continued to support the establishment of treatment and rehabilitation clinics in their communities. As much as possible, the chapters made social services available, including physical rehabilitation at home, occupational therapy, and transportation to clinics and meetings. Some chapters were more successful than others in providing services like these, but they all recognized the pressing needs of people with MS and became more aggressive in raising funds to expand the scope of their community outreach.

Meanwhile the National Society had outgrown its one-room office at the Academy of Medicine and moved its national headquarters to a suite of rooms at the Hotel Margery, a luxury apartment house at Park Avenue and 45th Street that had been scheduled for demolition. The Society paid only modest rent because of the Margery's short life expectancy, though the building stood for several more years because of postponements of its demise. But those headquarters—and a subsequent move to other offices on Park Avenue South—raised concerns among some Society supporters outside of New York who knew nothing about the inexpensive office space but suspected that a Park Avenue address was synonymous with living beyond one's means. "People thought we had lavish offices with carpets and drapes, but of course we had none of that," said Sylvia. "I constantly had to explain this away in meetings I had with the chapters."

In fact the Society made use of every corner and cubbyhole of its new offices. Dee Sammak, who began working for the Society in the 1950s, remembered fundraising canisters piled up in the Margery's bathtubs. "I can still picture myself in the bathroom, of all places, gathering canisters to pack them up and ship them to the chapters," she said. Dee recalls pitching in and doing whatever needed to be done, often under Sylvia's watchful eye. "As a young woman, I was frightened of her. She was such an imposing figure. But I soon came to see her as a warm and caring person. She was such an inspiration."

Straus had been less sure of Sylvia's role in the Society. He recruited Harry Murphy to assume her leadership position, but with an unfortunate outcome. Murphy had been national campaign director for the American Cancer Society, and Straus hoped he could stimulate the Society's fundraising. Murphy was given free rein and created a promotional idea that appealed to Straus: the Society would run a national contest in conjunction with a major beer manufacturer, the Rupert Brewery, placing receptacles in bars across the country. Bar customers were encouraged to write down the answer to a contest question, place it in an envelope—hopefully along with a contribution to the Society—and deposit it in the container.

The contest proved to be a bust. The bars did not collect much money, and the campaign died. In the process, according to Sylvia, Murphy made financial commitments that he had never been authorized to make. He had gambled on the contest's success, and the Society had lost. The organization was sued for $50,000 by a print shop. The case went to trial, but while the jury was deliberating, the Society's lawyers—against Sylvia's wishes—reached a settlement with the plaintiff, choosing to compromise rather than risk an adverse verdict. "Later, I spoke to a member of the jury, who told me that she and the rest of the panel had just come to a decision in our favor," Sylvia said. "I was shocked. I just couldn't deal with knowing that membership contributions would be wasted on an out-of-court settlement. It was one of the real heartbreaks of my life."

In the midst of this financial debacle, Ralph Straus accepted a government post overseas and left the Society. Before departing, he threw the budgetary crisis in Sylvia's lap. He told her, "I hope the Society is in existence when I get back."

Meanwhile, Murphy was dismissed. New staff members hired under Straus had to be laid off. Sylvia returned to her executive position, and her sister Alice gave up her job in order to work at the Society to help it recover. A crisis atmosphere persisted until the organization gradually extricated itself from its financial distress.

As a consequence of Murphy's fiasco the Society had few resources to support some of the research grants to which it was already committed. In desperation Sylvia met with Dr. Pearce Bailey, director of the federal government's National Institute for Neurological Diseases and Blindness, and appealed to him to take over the financing of these projects, which were highly regarded by the government's own peer-review committee. The National Society had always met its research-funding commitments and could have continued to do so were it not for the Rupert Brewery catastrophe. Because the society had maintained an excellent working relationship with Dr. Bailey, and because of the high quality of the Society's research, the Institute agreed to fund those studies. Nevertheless the shortfall was an embarrassment to the Society and an extremely stressful time for everyone involved.

Straus's prediction that top-level professional staff would not serve under a woman was not borne out. As the National MS Society's financial situation stabilized, Sylvia recruited professionals with impressive records of success in high-ranking positions in the voluntary health agency movement. Over the years, they included:

Dr. Harry Weaver, research director of the National Foundation for Infantile Paralysis (the Polio Foundation), who became the National MS Society's research director.

Wilbur Crawford, long-term assistant to Basil O'Connor at the National Foundation, who became Lawry's assistant.

Floyd Boyer, public relations director of the National Foundation, who became the National MS Society's public relations director.

Jess Speidel, national campaign director of the American Cancer Society, who became the National MS Society's national fundraising director.

James Walker, fundraising director of the Muscular Dystrophy Association, who became the National MS Society's fundraising director.

Years later Straus helped make amends. In 1973, after returning from his foreign assignment, he established the Ralph I. Straus Research Award—a Nobel-like prize to be awarded to the scientist or scientists, anywhere in the world, whose published research led to the development of an effective means of preventing and arresting MS. Straus made an initial grant of $100,000, which with interest and other contributions grew to a $1 million prize. When Straus announced the award at a news conference in Washington, D.C., he said, "I had always intended to leave a substantial bequest to the Society in my will. But after a recent discussion with scientists who told me of new leads developing in research, I decided to give the money now in the hope I might have the pleasure of hearing of the solution to MS while I am still alive."

The Society is still awaiting the breakthrough that will conquer the disease and make the awarding of that prize possible.

14

WHEN NANCY LONGSTRETH, a young Philadelphia homemaker, began experiencing double vision, slurred speech, and weakness in her extremities, she and her husband Thacher, who worked for *Life* magazine, were not prepared for what doctors told them. A neurologist at the University of Michigan Medical Center informed Thacher that his wife had multiple sclerosis. Thacher had never heard of the disease. The neurologist went on to paint a bleak picture of her future. "The doctors said that MS was going to kill her in a fairly short time—they gave her a life expectancy of another ten to fifteen years, with her condition deteriorating during that time," he recalled. They also advised Thacher not to tell his wife of her disease. "The news just destroyed me," said Thacher. "In our kitchen at home, I literally beat my head against the wall, trying to get the pain in my heart and in my brain balanced by the physical pain. I just didn't know what to do, and no one else seemed to either."

In the early 1950s Sylvia stressed the need to develop and disseminate information to people like Longstreth, as well as to professionals, through the Society's local chapters. It was a crucial part of the Society's growth. "Through conferences and the distribution of printed information, and reports in scientific publications, the medical profession is kept abreast of the newest developments and diagnostic methods and techniques of symptom management," she wrote in a Society report. "At the same time, the Society has been no less conscious of the need to combat the appalling ignorance and misconceptions that have surrounded multiple sclerosis since the disease first became known. To accomplish these objectives, comprehensive educational and public relations programs are considered the most important of the Society's responsibilities."

In 1952 the Society underwrote the publication of a series of manuals describing a home program of rehabilitation for all stages of the disease. Sylvia herself was the driving force behind these manuals because of her experience with Bernard's breakdown after his visit to the Kabat-Kaiser Institute. The content of the manuals was overseen by Dr. Howard Rusk, a well-known rehabilitation specialist, and the manuals were widely distributed to people with MS through their doctors, at no charge. "These manuals were used by many MS families and saved them a tremendous amount of money," said Sylvia. "Even when they couldn't afford professional therapy services, they could learn the right way to do it themselves from these manuals."

These materials took money to produce, and although the Society had raised money as aggressively as possible from its inception, it had never put together a coordinated national fund drive. Donations large and small were funneled into research projects. But as one doctor specializing in MS said, "A March of Dimes will never solve the problem of multiple sclerosis. It will take a March of Dollars."

In 1953 the Society launched its first national fundraising

appeal. Raymond Moley served as campaign chairman and oversaw a massive effort involving chapters and their volunteers in every part of the country. People dedicated to conquering MS walked through their neighborhoods and rang doorbells for the cause. Many thousands of people reached into their purses and pockets, donating dimes and dollars. The contributions reached record totals. The campaign demonstrated the strength of the chapters, which grew in each subsequent campaign. In 1955 the Society raised more than $1 million in a single year for the first time. High-profile Americans attached their names to the effort, led by Mamie Eisenhower, the First Lady, who served as honorary chairperson of the national drive for five years beginning in 1954. Entire organizations helped in the campaign, including the Veterans of Foreign Wars and its Ladies' Auxiliary—with a membership of 1.75 million.

During the mid-1950s one of the most prominent National Society spokespersons was Grace Kelly, who at that time was one of the most popular actresses in America. Before Prince Ranier entered her life, Kelly had been engaged to a young man—a friend of her brother's—who developed MS, and her commitment to conquering the disease arose from that relationship. She had been an active volunteer for the Philadelphia chapter, and then, at Sylvia's request, she agreed to become national campaign chairperson, a position she held for two years. During a reception in her honor at Gracie Mansion in New York, most of the male National Board members appeared to ignore her, not wanting to gawk at the beautiful movie star. Nevertheless Grace Kelly and Sylvia became friends in the years before she married Ranier and moved to Monaco. Soon after, Princess Grace and her husband issued a special stamp commemorating international research into MS supported by the National Society.

In 1954 the MS Key was chosen as the official symbol of the Society, shaped to open the doors that would ultimately solve the puzzle of this tragic disease. The MS Hope Chest also emerged in the 1950s as the theme of the Society's fundraising efforts. Tens of thousands of mail trucks throughout the country displayed campaign posters with slogans such as "There's No Vacation from MS." By 1957, contributions to the MS Hope Chest had escalated to $2.8 million.

The message about MS, and knowledge of the effort to find a cure, were finally reaching the American public.

15

WITH NO EFFECTIVE DRUGS and only limited techniques to ease the symptoms of MS, patients continued to seek miracles wherever possible. Doctors sometimes steered their patients toward treatments that were unproven but seemed to hold promise. One of these was the experimental use of ACTH, the natural pituitary gland secretion. ACTH had made its greatest impact as an anti-inflammatory treatment for people with arthritis. Grant money underwrote research and the testing of ACTH on people with MS. Dr. Cornelius Traeger, the Society's medical director, was particularly optimistic about the treatment's potential.

"If your brother Bernard were my sibling," he told Sylvia, "I'd take him by the hand and enroll him in our study of ACTH."

Sylvia convinced Bernard to try, and he participated in the study as an inpatient. The result, however, was catastrophic. "At the beginning of the study, Bernie was walking with a staggering gait, but he was still able to walk into the hospital," she said. "But when he came out of the hospital he was in a wheelchair for the first time. After close to a month of ACTH treatments, he never walked again."

Years later a clinical trial would show ACTH to be useful in some patients in reducing the intensity and duration of acute MS exacerbations. But after Bernard's disastrous experience with ACTH, Sylvia made a decision: "No more experiments for him." She was no longer willing to allow Bernard to become a test subject for unproven therapy. If he was going to be helped, it would be with treatments whose efficacy had been proven.

When faced with the diagnosis of multiple sclerosis, however, desperate people frequently fell prey to promoters of supposed cures they read of in the press or heard of through word of mouth. Some of these questionable treatments were touted by charlatans intent on exploiting vulnerable families. Others were championed by respected physicians who sincerely believed that they might be a source of genuine hope.

Thacher Longstreth heard about a controversial treatment being offered by a respected Detroit neurologist. It involved massive doses of penicillin, injected daily in the buttocks, intended to destroy bacteria that were purportedly causing or contributing to MS. "We decided to look into it for my wife," said Thacher. "We went to Michigan, met with the doctor, and he explained the treatment and showed me how to give the injections. I became quite good at giving the shots, and we did that for a couple of years. Her MS actually fared pretty well during that time, but she may have just been having a natural remission. I never really knew whether the treatment itself did much good."

In the early years of the Society, so-called cures being promoted in foreign countries were almost impossible to investigate. Claims filtered in from virtually every part of the world. Yet for the average person—and even for his or her physician—

there was nowhere to turn for authoritative information about a "breakthrough" drug or a "revolutionary" procedure. Grasping at straws, families mortgaged their homes or borrowed money from friends, and traveled thousands of miles in search of a miracle. Inevitably they ended up disappointed, sometimes destitute.

As Sylvia received phone calls and letters from people wiling to try just about any new treatment, she recognized the urgent need for reliable information about research and therapies. She brainstormed with Dr. Traeger. How could they investigate a treatment being offered by doctors in Moscow, Paris, or Madrid? Traeger decided to recruit a network of MS experts throughout the world, who could share information about research in their respective countries and assess experimental treatments there.

A committee of fifty-six leading neurologists from twenty-six countries became part of the International Panel of Corresponding Neurologists (which later evolved into the International Medical Advisory Board of the International Federation of Multiple Sclerosis Societies). They exchanged reports and shared ideas. They responded to questions from people with MS and their families. In the process they prevented many people from chasing false hopes. "When a person would inquire about a particular treatment being given to MS patients in a foreign country, we would turn to our representative in that country to provide a report to the Society's own Medical Advisory Board," said Sylvia. "In many cases we were able to put rumors and claims of cure to rest very quickly, before people had spent their life savings on them. Overall we probably saved MS families many millions of dollars."

The Panel of Corresponding Neurologists met for the first time in Lisbon in September 1953, during the International

Congress of Neurology, with both physicians and scientists attending. Its second meeting convened four years later, again as part of the International Congress of Neurology, this time in Brussels. Through the panel, the National Multiple Sclerosis Society became a worldwide clearinghouse of MS information—its first major step into the international arena. In the process, Sylvia gradually recognized that the National Society could not ignore the global character of the disease and the leadership role it could play in stimulating research throughout the world. "I felt strongly that by encouraging scientists overseas to study MS, we would hasten the day of finding the answer," she said. Later, in the 1960s, the Society played a crucial role in the creation of an international body to promote research and services for people with MS everywhere.

As far-reaching and effective as the Society had become as it approached its tenth anniversary, it still could not cite any major breakthroughs in the fight against MS. This was acutely frustrating given the dynamic advances in medicine in the 1950s. The pacemaker saved the lives of many people with heart disease. The first open-heart surgeries were performed. Tuberculosis was treated effectively for the first time. The Salk vaccine rescued children from the ravages of polio. Effective treatments for MS, however, remained elusive.

Yet the Society had dramatically changed the environment for MS patients and their families. The disease was more widely recognized and taken much more seriously by the medical community than ever before. Fewer doctors were misdiagnosing MS or dismissing people with the disease as being "crazy" or "hysterical," or as having suffered a stroke. Interest among outstanding scientists in conducting MS research increased dramatically. In 1955 the Society's annual report boldly stated, "We can envisage the day when multiple sclerosis no longer spreads its blight over the nation and the world." MS Hope Chest funds supported studies at the most respected and prestigious scientific centers in the country—Albert Einstein College of Medicine in New York, the Harvard Medical School, UCLA Medical Center, the University of Michigan Medical Center, Philadelphia General Hospital—as well as a growing number of institutions abroad (including the University of Alberta in Canada and University Hospital in Hamburg, Germany). By 1955 the Society had raised and committed more than $1 million for MS research—a momentous achievement for a new organization. By the end of the decade, 117 projects had been approved by the Medical Advisory Board.

At Washington University Medical School, researchers studied the biochemical components of central nervous system tissue, which they hoped would shed light on the chemical structure of myelin.

At Albert Einstein College of Medicine, scientists investigated the mechanism by which myelin is formed in the central nervous system.

At the Neurological Clinic, University of Hamburg, tissue culture methods were used to study the possible effects of MS on certain chemical components of the blood.

At Georgetown University School of Medicine, investigators explored the precise chemical composition of spinal fluid and how it might be altered by MS.

At Indiana University School of Medicine, scientists studied nerve lesions in mice that developed after exposure to viruses. Though these researchers did not contend that a virus was responsible for MS, they believed that it was a way to study degeneration of the myelin sheath.

In an epidemiological study by Mayo Clinic researchers, MS was found to be more common in countries distant from the equator, a curious pattern that soon became the focus of much more investigation. Surveys found a higher prevalence of MS in the northern United States than in the southern regions; this same phenomenon was observed in Europe as well.

One of the most intriguing MS studies of this era was conceived by Oliver Buckley, who had become vice president of the National Society in the early 1950s. Buckley was chairman of Bell Telephone Laboratories, the largest industrial research corporation in the country. Trained as an engineer, he was widely known for his pioneering work on high-speed telegraph cables. Buckley became involved in the National Society after reading an article on MS in the *New York Times* while stuck in his limousine in Manhattan traffic. He ordered his driver to change their route and head for the Society's office. He arrived without an appointment, with the newspaper article in his hand. He introduced himself to Sylvia and said, "From the description of multiple sclerosis that appears in this article, I have a strong suspicion that my son has been misdiagnosed, and that he actually has MS." Buckley asked penetrating questions and wanted copies of the Society's literature to read. "Before the end of our meeting," Sylvia recalled, "he had decided to consult a neurologist about his son's condition."

Within two weeks, Buckley's son had been diagnosed with MS. Buckley then volunteered his time and influence to the Society, and soon became a member of the Board of Directors. He addressed himself to strengthening the Society's leadership and applied his business acumen to the internal workings of the organization. Buckley had credited his own success in corporate America not to any particular personal brilliance or genius but to his ability to surround himself with the most capable people he could find. He urged Sylvia to do the same. "When recruiting your staff, don't reject a person who might be a threat to you because he's too strong," he told her. "Go after the strongest staff members you can find, because they will only add to your own effectiveness." As Buckley's own commitment to the Society strengthened with time, he told Sylvia, "Whenever you need me—day or night, on the weekends, even when I'm traveling abroad on business—contact my secretary and she will reach me, wherever I am."

Because of Buckley's scientific background—he was the first chairman of the Science Advisory Committee of President Truman's Office of Defense Mobilization, and had been a member of the Atomic Energy Commission's advisory panel—he took a particular interest in the research directions of the National Multiple Sclerosis Society. At Bell Laboratories, when faced with technical problems, he had relied on the art of brainstorming. He invited the best scientific minds to address a particular problem, bringing them together in an informal, relaxed setting where they could exchange ideas that often led to concrete advances. Buckley introduced the same concept to the National Society. At his urging, the organization assembled a small group of the country's top neuroscientists and encouraged them to brainstorm about MS research and where it should be heading. Dr. Harold Wainerdi, who succeeded Dr. Cornelius Traeger as the Society's medical director, coordinated and led these meetings. New ideas and even grant applications grew out of the sessions.

One of the best ideas was proposed by Buckley himself. The roles of genetics and environment in MS had piqued his interest, and he developed the concept of a study involving twins—one twin with MS, the other without. "Every element of their backgrounds and their lives could be studied to try to determine what may have contributed to the development of MS in one of them, and what might have protected the other," he said. The Medical Advisory Board was intrigued with the idea, and Dr. Roland Mackay was awarded a grant to conduct the research, which was undertaken primarily at the University of Illinois and the University of Minnesota. The Society asked its chapters to look for twins in their communities who would be willing to participate.

For five years Dr. Mackay studied 34 pairs of identical twins and 26 pairs of fraternal twins, one or both of whom had MS. His conclusion: "There is probably a genetically transmitted vulnerability to MS in the patients studied. Agents from outside the body more readily attack those with a predisposing hereditary element, an element that seems unable to produce disease by itself." Dr. Mackay was also able to examine the health records of 2,900 close and distant relatives of the twins in his study. He reported, "In every category of relationship, the prevalence of multiple sclerosis is many times that found in the total population. And the closer the relationship, the higher the prevalence of MS."

Oliver Buckley ultimately developed Parkinson's disease, and died in 1959. His wife, Clara, said that when he was lapsing into and out of a coma before his death, he was whispering to himself about the problems confronting the National MS Society. "The affairs of the Society had gripped him so much that he worried about the plight of MS patients night and day," said Sylvia. For decades after Buckley's death, Sylvia was guided by his advice, including his emphasis on the importance of surrounding oneself with the most competent people available.

Oliver Buckley's commitment to research became a major impetus behind advancements in the scientific understanding of MS. When Dr. Thomas Willmon was appointed the Society's medical director in 1956, he spoke about research developments at a regional conference and pointed to many areas of progress. "One of the most interesting and hopeful developments is the ability to grow successfully and reliably central nervous system cells in tissue culture—that is, the growth of brain tissue in test tubes," Willmon said. "The techniques allow not only the growth of these delicate cells but also continuous observation of their development and even the formation and destruction of myelin. . . . It is hoped that this technique can be used for delineation of many unknowns about brain tissue, myelin, and favorable or unfavorable influences which may exert themselves upon its metabolism."

For every step forward, however, there also were disappointments. At the Jewish Sanitarium and Hospital for Chronic Diseases in New York City, scientists thought that the analysis of protein changes in the blood of people with MS might provide a means for diagnosing the disease, but this approach did not materialize. Neither did another possible diagnostic marker. At the University of Rochester, cyanide had been observed in people with MS, and for a time there was hope that its presence might be an indicator of multiple sclerosis.

In the late 1950s, to accelerate progress on the scientific front, the National Society awarded its first fellowships to support the training of young MS researchers. It also established the Central Registry of Pathological Material at New York's Montefiore Hospital. The registry became the depository of the nation's largest collection of brains, spinal cords, and peripheral nerves from deceased people with MS; when investigators and medical centers conducting research into the disease needed tissue and other material, they turned to the registry.

As the years passed, scientists acknowledged that multiple sclerosis was much more complex than they had once believed, and that conquering it was a monumental challenge. Doctors had begun to utilize a status scale, refined by Dr. John Kurtzke, to help determine disability levels and the portions of the nervous system affected by MS. But effective treatments and the ultimate answer were still distant. At the close of the 1950s, Dr. Willmon observed, "If it were yet possible to pinpoint the scientific area from which the solution will be found, the research could and should be concentrated, even saturated in that area. But there are as yet many possibilities, and there are so many basic facts which need to be known in order to understand the mechanics and mechanisms of the brain and nervous system which are involved in multiple sclerosis that a broad and frontal attack on the problem continues to be necessary."

Willmon added, "I think we now have three big obvious clues, the solution to any one of which might well open the door to learning the cause of multiple sclerosis. One is the fact that the great majority of cases are diagnosed between the ages of twenty and forty. Another is the disparity in geographic distribution. And the third is the fact that a patient with multiple sclerosis, so disabled that he is unable to get out of his bed or wheelchair, may within a period of a few days or weeks be walking. How this dramatic type of remission happens, what change occurs in the body chemically or otherwise to enable the patient to function, must certainly hold a lead to the answer. When any or all of these clues are broken, we will truly have made progress."

Even as research intensified, the pressures for answers grew, giving rise to conflicts within the Society. Dr. Willmon had previously been director of research for the U.S. Navy and had been more of an administrator than a bench scientist. While Sylvia and certain members of the Medical Advisory Board supported research following up on the specific clues that were emerging from Society-funded research, Dr. Willmon insisted, "There is still a lot of basic, fundamental research in neurology that needs to be done. We can't influence science. We've got to give the researchers the money and let them run with it." Sylvia remembered that Willmon thought she was "off the beam" when she pushed for a planned or targeted research program while he insisted that research should follow a more fundamental, serendipitous course that would give investigators free rein. Ultimately she won the support of Dr. H. Houston Merritt, vice chairman of the Medical Advisory Board, and then that of the Medical Board and the Board of Directors. A Research Evaluation and Planning Committee was appointed. Soon thereafter, a disappointed Dr. Willmon resigned his position.

16

IN 1952 the MS Society could count seventy-nine chapters and branches across the nation, each with members dedicated to advancing research, patient care, and education. As the decade progressed, more chapters were established, usually due to volunteers like Thacher Longstreth. When Thacher traveled on business, he asked the national staff for a list of Society members in the cities where he was headed, and sent letters or made phone calls in advance, inviting people there to attend a chapter-planning meeting at the hotel where he would be staying. By encouraging participation this way, Thacher stimulated the creation of chapters in Jacksonville, Atlanta, Buffalo, Rochester, Pittsburgh, Washington, D.C., and other cities.

The chapters became the backbone of the Society. They helped establish and support MS clinics and evaluation centers, which had increased to twenty-seven in number by the mid-1950s. The chapters also provided home-care assistance for families and supported public education programs, including the distribution of thousands of copies of the brochure "What

Is MS?" Some began providing equipment loans for people with MS; others launched recreational and social programs. As much as anything, these local organizations renewed hope and dignity to people with MS, and helped them feel less isolated in their own communities.

On the national level, key individuals moved the Society forward. William Breed was head of the New York law firm of Breed, Abbott & Morgan. His son Alan had MS. When the *New York Times* published the first article on the new national organization in 1946, Breed phoned Carl Owen and offered to help the Society in any way he could. Most important, he encouraged his other son, William Jr., to join the national board and eventually serve as its chairman beginning in the mid-1950s. William Breed, Jr., was also an attorney in his father's firm. He possessed great organizational skills, and like Sylvia Lawry soon considered the Society's mission to be his own and dedicated himself to finding the cure for MS. He opened every board meeting by turning to the Society's medical director, and asking, "Have you found a cure yet?" It was a rhetorical question, but he believed it reinforced the reason why they had gathered there and the importance of what they were trying to accomplish.

When Breed spoke at public meetings, he began by talking of his brother's struggle with the disease. Tears often rolled down his cheeks. He once related the story of Alan losing his equilibrium at a large gathering of people, and sprawling on the floor. Breed told the group, "I'll never forget the way Alan reacted. A big smile came over his face, and he made fun of his 'clumsiness.' He put everyone else at ease."

Thacher Longstreth said of Breed, "Bill Breed was a heck of a guy. Next to Sylvia Lawry, he probably had a greater impact on the national organization than anyone I knew."

While people like Breed worked tirelessly in the trenches, the Society continued to involve celebrities to help give it the increased public visibility it needed. Robert Montgomery served as campaign chairman. Walter Pidgeon, Rosalind Russell, Irene Dunne, Greer Garson, Sammy Kaye, Rock Hudson, Ed Sullivan, and many others recorded announcements for the MS Hope Chest Campaign. Pat Boone headed Teens Against MS. Guy Lombardo chaired Musicians Against MS. Polly Bergen lent her name to the Women's Activities Committee. Mel Allen served as chairman of Good Sports for MS and promoted the MS Hope Chest on 154 Yankee broadcasts in 1958. In years to come, celebrities such as Paul Newman, Barbra Streisand, Julie Andrews, and many others lent their names and talent to the ranks of those fighting the disease.

The most inspired commitment, however, came from those whose lives and families had been directly touched by multiple sclerosis. That was the case with Shirley Temple Black. During the 1930s, Shirley Temple had achieved greater motion picture popularity than any child actor since Jackie Coogan. But her storybook personal life was shattered when her brother George was diagnosed with MS. A survivor of the attack on Pearl Harbor, George had suffered a stroke in the early 1950s. While he was recovering, Dr. Augustus Rose, a UCLA neurologist and member of the Society's Medical Advisory Board, diagnosed him as also having MS.

At that point Shirley Temple Black began volunteering at the chapter in Los Angeles. When she was elected to the National Board of Directors in 1958, and was appointed national chair of volunteers, she spearheaded the society's fundraising efforts. Later she played a key role in the development of the international MS movement. "Without Miss Black's involvement, we probably never would have had an international federation," said Charles W. V. (Vic) Meares. Meares, who became the National Society's vice president in 1958, knew something about the role celebrities could play in fighting MS: Meares had been attracted to helping the Society after hearing a speech by Dr. Harold Wainerdi, then the Society's associate medical director. "I was very moved by what I heard," said Meares. "I felt that it was bad enough for people to be afflicted with MS, but no one was paying much attention to them, and that seemed a dreadful thing to me. So I felt more impelled to do something about MS than about anything I'd ever done before. Most of the people active in the Society had their families touched by MS, but I came to believe that the best efforts of the organization should be carried by those of us who have been fortunate enough not to have direct family involvement with the disease. It's enough to have MS in your family without also having to go out on evenings and weekends, raising money or doing other things to support the cause."

Meares, vice president and later chairman of the board of the New York Life Insurance Company, was often described as the most respected executive in the insurance industry. When Joan Crawford and her husband, Alfred Steele, president of Pepsi-Cola, offered themselves to the cause, Meares and Sylvia Lawry went to their Fifth Avenue apartment to discuss the ways in which Miss Crawford might become active.

"We were met at the door by a maid, who asked us to take off our shoes before we entered," said Meares. "She said that Miss Crawford did not like shoes touching her carpets. Well, for some reason, I refused! After a few uncomfortable moments, she invited us in anyway. Once inside, I could see why the request had been made. The carpets were totally white. So was all of the furniture. Interestingly, several months later, Joan told me that one of the reasons she admired me was that I was the only person who had ever refused to take his shoes off at her doorstep!"

In 1957, Crawford narrated "In Sickness and Health," a thirty-minute film produced by the National MS Society. It was broadcast on thirty television stations around the country. Later, when Crawford agreed to serve as national campaign chairperson for the Society, Meares met with her several more times, including a visit to her mansion in the Brentwood area of Los Angeles. He arrived promptly at 2:30 on a Saturday afternoon and rang the doorbell repeatedly, without getting a response. Finally the door opened, and he was greeted by Crawford's teenage daughter, Christina. She had obviously been crying, and her eyes were still brimming with tears. "Please come in and go to the living room," she said. "My mother will be with you in a while."

Later, Meares said, "Joan told me that Christina had been a bad girl, was being punished, and that the chauffeur was taking her back to boarding school rather than allowing her to attend a party that evening. I don't know what Christina was being punished for. But that was how I met the author of *Mommie Dearest*."

17

IN THE SHADOW of her work with the Society and its growing national presence, Sylvia still attended to Bernard, the person who had motivated her from the start. Bernard was typical of an individual with ever-increasing needs due to the chronic, progressive nature of his disease. When Bernard's vision began to fail, Sylvia prevailed upon the Library of Congress (specifically, its Division for the Blind and Physically Handicapped) to make "talking books" available to individuals with MS. The Society's chapters helped distribute thousands of phonographs to people with MS, and helped disseminate a wide range of "reading" material, including the classics, current and popular fiction and nonfiction, and many magazines. Overnight, individuals unable to read because of poor eyesight or the inability to hold a book or turn its pages could enjoy "reading." Before long the Telephone Pioneers, an association of employees of AT&T, agreed to repair the phonographs of MS patients without charge.

Though Bernard's condition gradually worsened, he actually became more hopeful about his fate. As Sylvia told him that researchers were making progress, Bernard began to plan a future for himself. He was willing to seriously consider marriage for the first time.

Sylvia's sister Alice had befriended a co-worker named Teresa, a vivacious, outgoing woman with a wonderful sense of humor. She introduced Bernard to Teresa, and from their first meeting there was clearly a chemistry between them. When they began to discuss marriage, Sylvia and Alice were delighted. Sylvia sat down with Teresa, however, and fully explained Bernard's illness. She also asked her physician to talk with Teresa to ensure that she knew that her future husband's physical condition might deteriorate. Bernard became fatigued easily and lived a largely sedentary life. Although he couldn't work, his father offered to support the couple if they married. Teresa understood that their future was uncertain, but she decided to marry Bernard.

After the couple's wedding, Sylvia moved out of the home that she had shared with Bernard, and she and Alice rented an apartment in New York City. About two years later, Bernard and his wife had a son. Bernard was overjoyed. Years earlier he had worried that MS might make him impotent and keep him from ever having children. But Sylvia came up with what was then a truly novel idea. "Bernie," she told him, "we'll freeze your sperm and then use it when you want to have children." There were no sperm banks in those days, but she approached Dr. Wainerdi with the idea. He initially thought it was rather odd. Nevertheless he agreed to arrange for the sperm to be frozen and stored. In the end, Bernard never had to use it; his son was conceived naturally. Meanwhile, Sylvia married Stanley Englander, and before long they had two sons, Steven and Frank. For both Bernard and Sylvia, a sense of contentment came to their personal lives.

With his own wife and child, Bernard was the happiest he had been in a very long time. But his happiness didn't last long. When Teresa looked into the future, she felt insecure and saw little promise that his condition would improve. Soon after the birth of their son, the marriage began to dissolve. Teresa walked out, moving to Brooklyn and taking their son with her.

Bernard was devastated. He tried to see his son as often as possible, and his sister Lillian drove him to Brooklyn a number of times. But Teresa finally said, "No more visits!" He eventually lost contact with his son. For Bernard, it was a crueler blow than even multiple sclerosis. "Bernie would ask me to try to get in touch with them and arrange for the child to visit him," said Sylvia, who moved back in with Bernard after his marriage collapsed. "But Teresa wouldn't agree, and I was told that the boy didn't want to see his father. I couldn't tell Bernie that, so I pretended that I was too busy to make the contact. I told Bernie, 'I'll get to it in a few weeks.' It was so heartbreaking for him."

Such problems are not uncommon among families with MS. The family unit is placed under enormous pressure. It can be disrupted and undermined. It can also remain united and strong. When the wife of Charles Steifel, a Chicago attorney, was diagnosed with MS, he went to great lengths to maintain normalcy in the family and to keep his spouse as a full, active member of the family. When Sylvia Lawry visited them in their home, at a time when Mrs. Steifel was bedridden, Charles had permanently placed her bed in the living room so that she could be part of the events when they socialized. Sylvia was particularly touched by this gesture that the family made to ensure that Mrs. Steifel lived life to the fullest. "For the person with MS to survive emotionally, he or she needs the support of the family," Sylvia said.

The Society's 1959 Annual Report honored the thousands

of people who had struggled with private traumas and yet had given time and contributions to the organization: "In gratitude for progress in the present and the vision of success in the future, this Annual Report is dedicated to the MS volunteer—to the homemakers, the wage earners, the doctors, the lawyers, the businessmen, the industrialists, the patients and their families—to all who so freely and generously give their time, energy, skill, and resources to the humanitarian partnership of the National Multiple Sclerosis Society."

18

THE 1960s was one of America's most turbulent decades. A young, charismatic president was elected, and three years later he was assassinated. Civil rights activists rallied against injustice, and anti-war demonstrators shouted their grievances on the streets of every major city. On the medical front, the surgeon general spoke out about the risks of cigarette smoking. Dr. Christiaan Barnard performed the first heart transplant. Millions of women began using the birth-control pill. In this environment, the MS movement faced the challenge of conquering a disease that had proven to be a particularly formidable adversary.

The National Multiple Sclerosis Society launched the decade with the 1960 Hope Chest Campaign slogan: "Home Is Where the Hurt Is—When MS Hits." Two years later, another slogan captured the imagination of volunteers and contributors: "WHEN Will MS Be Cured? . . . Say WHEN with Your Dollars." As the National Society's 1962 Annual Report declared, those waging the war against MS viewed the organization's mission as a "challenge to man's social responsibility . . . a claim on his conscience. In the perspective of history, it is man joining together with man to improve welfare . . . to advocate human knowledge and well-being."

President John F. Kennedy became the most prominent booster of the battle against MS. While still a U.S. senator he had become campaign chairman of the Society's Massachusetts chapter, and then national campaign chairman. JFK had a personal interest in the disease. His cousin Ann Gargan had MS, and despite her own illness, she had become a constant caretaker of the president's father, Joseph P. Kennedy, after he suffered a stroke in 1961. As president, John Kennedy continued his active interest in multiple sclerosis. At one point he suggested to Sylvia Lawry that he would host a press conference at the White House, in which one of the leading scientists in the field would talk about research developments in MS and introduce more of the nation to the disease. Dr. Murray B. Bornstein of Albert Einstein College of Medicine and a recipient of a Society research grant was chosen to join Kennedy at that White House gathering. It was a huge success.

Behind the scenes in the 1960s, the staff and volunteers at the national headquarters and the chapter offices confronted enormous and sometimes overwhelming challenges. The problems of every person with multiple sclerosis became their own. Every MS family's plight heightened their own dedication. The National MS Society's commitment to research accelerated, and the Society funded a committee of experts headed by Dr. George Schumacher to create criteria for the diagnosis of MS. These standards (with refinements) are still used today and have significantly minimized the problem of misdiagnosis of MS.

The ongoing work at the chapter level continued to inspire everyone in the movement. There were 114 chapters by

1960, and some of them joined forces with the American Red Cross to increase their capacity to provide home nursing and transportation for people with MS. The number of people assisted by local service programs soared 50 percent in the early 1960s. In 1963 alone, chapter staff and volunteers made approximately 24,000 visits to people with MS; 28,000 individuals with the disease received physical or occupational therapy; 26,000 used clinics or medically directed outpatient services; 16,400 were subsidized in obtaining visiting nursing services; 23,000 were loaned equipment and aids to daily living; and 46,000 participated in recreational activities. It was an impressive record.

These efforts helped people like Rosemary Pixley, a courageous mother living with the disease. In the 1960s, when Rosemary was featured in an article in *MS Keynotes*, a National Society publication, she described how important the Society had been to her. She expressed her gratitude for an elaborate $256 wheelchair donated by the St. Louis Area Chapter of the Society. "I wear out wheelchairs the way other people wear out shoes," she said. To repay the kindness, she spent many hours each week on the phone, and recruited two hundred house-to-house fundraisers in her neighborhood. She described her husband, Charlie, as her strength, and worried more about him than herself. "He has to be my hands, my legs," she said. "He never has any time off. He doesn't like housework, but he goes ahead and does it anyway. I don't think I'd be as tolerant of him if this situation were reversed. I take everything out on him. I know how lucky I am—not everybody has a Charlie."

One of Rosemary Pixley's neighbors—a divorced mother of four—had MS that had progressed so rapidly that she could no longer feed herself. She described living on welfare and relying on her children to care for her in relays. Her college-age son did the marketing, her twelve-year-old daughter prepared breakfast, her ten-year-old son came home from school to make lunch, and her fourteen-year-old son fixed dinner. The chapter provided her with a $220 hospital bed and a costly hydraulic lift that helped her move into her wheelchair. As she said, "I would never have been able to cope with this handicap if it weren't for my children and the National Multiple Sclerosis Society." When she was asked what she dreamed of more than anything, she whispered, "I just wish someone would find a cure for this."

That continued to be Sylvia Lawry's dream. "Sylvia was absolutely amazing during those days," said Thacher Longstreth. "The organization was growing, both nationally and locally, and she still was handling so much herself, working hundred-hour weeks. With time, by necessity, she became a little better at delegating responsibility, and she used some of us to handle problems in the field on the chapter level. My phone would ring and it would be Sylvia, asking me to go to a particular city to resolve a problem or come to New York for a special meeting—and I'd always do it. My wife used to joke that she didn't know whether I was married to her or to Sylvia and the Society. But a lot of us almost worshipped Sylvia because of her personal strength and the manner in which she sacrificed everything in her life for this organization. She gave me hope, and she showed me the basic toughness and tenacity that I needed in order to do what was necessary. You don't meet many people like that in your lifetime."

Despite the Society's successes, periodic mini-crises did arise from time to time at the chapter level. Charles (Vic) Meares was part of Lawry's informal team of "firefighters"—all of whom were members of the national board—who would fan out across the country and smother the brush fires that would occasionally flare at the chapters. Meares spent decades as a volunteer, serving as vice president and national campaign chairman. Sylvia called him "the power behind the throne," insisting that "no significant move was ever made by a Society president without first consulting Vic Meares. Vic said that when he first came on the board he was very unsure about me; but it didn't take him long to realize that I knew what I was doing."

When Meares was chairman of the Chapter Relations Committee, he tried to quiet any storms at the local level— most often rebellions against the formula that divided funds between chapters and the national office. "Of course the National Society wanted its share for research," said Meares, "but the local chapters had patients on their doorsteps who needed things like wheelchairs and transportation to clinics. Sylvia strongly believed that research should remain the top agenda item while also recognizing the practicality of providing local services, and that in order for local people to donate money, you've got to do something for them locally."

All major voluntary health agencies have conflicts over how funds should be spent, but with multiple sclerosis, in which people so often have immediate and pressing needs, some chapter officials have always cringed at the thought of spending money on anything other than urgent patient services in their own communities. While many of the chapters had become excellent fundraisers, others had fallen into debt and flinched at the idea of sending 40 percent of the funds they raised to the national headquarters. When the tremors of chapter rebellion were felt all the way back to New York, Sylvia often hit the road herself, traveling from one city to another, turning her briefcase into a portable office, running the national headquarters from hotel phones in one city or another.

At times the only solution she saw was to move an ineffective chapter's executive director into early retirement, though she had to lobby the local board members to take that kind of action. "It was a very trying period," she said. "Sometimes the right people weren't there to raise the kinds of funds that were needed. So, working from my hotel room, I'd have to get certain people ousted and move the right people into positions of local influence."

At one point, many of the chapters in the major cities—including Los Angeles, Baltimore, Washington, D.C., and the Boston area—threatened to withdraw from the National MS Society and form their own splinter organization unless the 60–40 split were changed. They insisted that they could not meet their local expenses with the existing formula. Sylvia traveled from one city to the next, quieting the rebellion. She often explained—and then reexplained—that there was nothing wrong with the 60–40 formula for the division of funds. The chapters simply had to work harder at raising more money if there wasn't enough to support their local programs. "The public contributes on the basis of the 60–40 split, and we can't go against that pledge to them," she told chapter representatives. She often arrived at local offices with concrete ideas for fundraising, such as house-to-house campaigns with support from the national staff. When the National Society created a highly publicized honor roll of chapters that donated in excess of the usual formula, allocating a higher percentage for research, some local officials clamored to climb aboard that bandwagon.

"The chapters raising the money wanted research to go forward, but they had their own important projects too," said Meares. "So while I totally agreed with Sylvia in principle, I tried to tell her that at times you had to be a good compromiser. She and I had some of our sharpest disagreements over this issue, though even as we argued, I never lost sight of her extraordinary and single-minded devotion to this cause."

The national headquarters recognized how crucial the chapters were to the movement, and felt that some were doing a superb job. But the national board still believed that it needed to intervene at times. On one occasion, at Sylvia's request, Palmer Brown and Alida Camp traveled to Florida to inform officials of the Miami chapter that their charter was being revoked because they were doing such a poor job of recruiting good leadership and raising money. "Initially they had no idea why we were there, and just figured that we had come to pay them a visit," said Brown. "They greeted us with open arms and smiles, and told us how delighted they were to welcome members of the national board. Then, when we told them that we were there to cancel their charter, you could hear a pin drop."

Despite such inevitable conflicts, the chapters proved their worth, day after day, providing a resource in the community to meet people's needs. "So often I would get a phone call from someone with multiple sclerosis, and I'd listen to him for fifteen minutes, and before we'd hang up, he'd say something like, 'Thank you, you've helped me so much,'" said Thacher Longstreth. "But during the call, I had barely said anything. I had just listened. That is exactly what many MS patients need—someone to listen with a sympathetic ear."

The chapters were also the training ground for many of the Society's most skilled leaders. Norman Cohn was one of the best. A tall, gentle-voiced executive in the Chicago construction industry, Cohn's wife was diagnosed with multiple sclerosis in 1958. Before long he became a member and then chairman of the Chicago chapter's board of trustees. In the 1960s he joined the Society's national Board of Directors and became one of its most enthusiastic and dedicated members while remaining a driving force with the Chicago chapter. Before long, Cohn had risen to the vice presidency, then the presidency and the chairmanship of the National Society, where he placed a great emphasis on maximizing volunteer involvement. He created a structure—specifically, the regional councils—to facilitate contact and communication between national and chapter volunteers. He also invited three to four chapter chairmen to each national board meeting, and took steps to expand patient programs and MS research.

When the National Society dedicated its 1981 annual report to Cohn, it proclaimed, "This 6'3" man—who stands 9' tall among those who know him—has contributed his time, wisdom and personal resources in enormously generous amounts. . . . He has brought to each and every undertaking a freshness and clarity of view, a sensitivity and generosity of spirit, and a set of professional skills that has left an indelible stamp on the Society." Cohn's commitment to the National Multiple Sclerosis Society continued years after his death. In his will he left $2 million for MS research. His battle against multiple sclerosis goes on in laboratories in many parts of the country.

19

IN THE COMMUNITIES with multiple sclerosis clinics, people had a place to turn for excellent care. One of those Society-affiliated facilities was operated by Dr. Leo Alexander, a prominent Boston neurologist with a strong commitment to people with MS. He had received a number of National Society grants to conduct clinical research at Boston State Hospital. But when Dr. Alexander's grants came up for renewal, the National Society's Medical Advisory Board raised skeptical eyebrows about the direction of his research. One board member remarked, "He's been on a fishing expedition for so long, and it hasn't borne out any significant developments. His grant application is too vague and general." The board voted to reject his latest application for additional funds.

The decision infuriated Dr. Alexander. But rather than accept the judgment, he turned to an unlikely source for research money—the Boston chapter of the Society. This maneuver was clearly a violation of national policy, which placed the responsibility for research funding decisions upon the national Medical Advisory Board and the national Board of

Directors. Yet the Boston chapter appropriated funds for Dr. Alexander's research in violation of national policy, risking the revocation of its charter.

Sylvia was taken aback by Dr. Alexander's strategy, which had sidestepped the Society's approved channels for research support. Alexander was a member of the very Medical Advisory Board that had rejected his grant application, and he knew the Society's policy well. A schism immediately developed between the National Society and the local chapter, where Alexander had some strong support, including the backing of the newly appointed chapter chairman. Frantic, principally because of the precedent it might set for other chapters, Sylvia caught a train for Boston to try to calm tensions and prevent a chapter revolt. As soon as she arrived at her hotel, the phone in her room rang. "It was Dr. Alexander, and he threatened me. 'If you value your health,' he said, 'you'll get out of Boston on the next train.' His voice was highly charged, and I became quite distressed," Sylvia recalled. "I'm sure he wasn't going to cause me physical harm, but I was disturbed at how angry he was. He knew why I was there, and he clearly wanted me out of Boston."

Mary Cohn, an influential force in the Boston chapter and a member of the national and chapter boards, came to Sylvia's defense. Cohn and her husband owned toy and plastics companies, and she had traveled the world to find help for her son with MS. She believed that since the national Medical Advisory Board had turned down Dr. Alexander's grant application, there was no reason to consider funding it on the local level. She gradually persuaded a number of local board members to support her point of view, but there was still plenty of local opposition to this intrusion by the national headquarters. Dr. Alexander was spreading the word in the MS community and among scientists in Boston that the national office was trying to "destroy" his clinic. As a result, a groundswell of support for Alexander grew among Boston's neurologists, some of whom told Sylvia that they would stand behind their colleague. A game of political maneuvering was under way, and at least for the moment, it was a stalemate.

Sylvia called Dr. H. Houston Merritt, vice chairman of the national Medical Advisory Board, who had been a professor of neurology at the Harvard Medical School before moving to the Neurological Institute in New York to become its director. "Here I am, trying to enforce the decision that your Medical Advisory Board has reached, and it's becoming a real nightmare," Sylvia told him. Merritt listened quietly, then said, "I'm going to try to help you." He placed a call to Dr. Joseph Foley, a respected neurologist at Boston City Hospital, and asked him to meet with Sylvia. Foley agreed, became convinced that Sylvia's position was correct, and said he would openly support her. In just days Foley had changed the entire tenor of the debate. One by one, local neurologists moved over to the side of the National Society. Even so, some members of the chapter remained steadfast in their revolt. The battle raged. The wounds festered.

As Sylvia's frustration escalated, Mary Cohn referred her to a high-profile Boston civil attorney, Claude Cross, who had represented Alger Hiss years earlier. As they planned strategy together, they decided to take up the matter at the chapter's upcoming annual meeting, where new members of the board would be elected and the matter could be debated. In anticipation of that showdown, Dr. Alexander contacted dozens of his MS patients in Boston and persuaded them to attend the meeting and vote against those board candidates supporting the national office's effort to "destroy my clinic." He even collected proxy votes from people who couldn't travel to attend the meeting. At the same time the anti-Alexander forces were building their own momentum, including signing up new members of the Society who had pro-Lawry sentiments. In addition, questions were now being raised as to whether it was appropriate to operate an MS clinic in a mental hospital.

When the annual meeting was finally gaveled into session, both sides argued their positions passionately. The debate was intense, loud, emotional, and exhausting. At times it almost took on the aura of a life-and-death struggle. Many members became disturbed by the heated division within the organization. When the vote was finally taken, the pro–National Society forces had prevailed, and the bylaws that prohibited chapter-financed research were reaffirmed. The vote wasn't close. Sylvia had won the day. Looking back, some of those who witnessed the proceedings thought it was a hallmark event in the voluntary health movement.

"Of course, my goal was never to destroy Dr. Alexander's clinic but to remove chapter-funded research from its program," said Sylvia. "I was only trying to enforce national policy that I believed in. In the heat of the battle, and amid all of the maneuvering, Dr. Alexander managed to foresee nearly every move I made, and he was very good at developing strategies for circumventing what I was trying to do. There were many nights I didn't sleep, taking one hot bath after another, trying to calm myself and figure out how to resolve this matter. It was one of the most stressful times in the history of the Society."

A reconstituted chapter board in Boston immediately affiliated itself with a treatment clinic divorced from research. Clinical services for persons with MS were not interrupted.

20

SYLVIA LAWRY never vacationed like most people do. Instead of packing her suitcase with suntan lotion and tour books, she filled it with multiple sclerosis literature and a list of contacts who might help the movement. That included her trips abroad, where she paid her own way to offer encouragement and comfort to people with multiple sclerosis and guide them in launching MS societies in their own countries.

Those countless meetings and tens of thousands of miles of travel ultimately produced the International Federation of Multiple Sclerosis Societies, formally founded in 1967. But the groundwork for that historic event spanned many years, with its seeds planted as early as 1948. From the beginning of the National Society, Sylvia sensed the need eventually to spread the movement globally. Whenever letters arrived at the New York office from abroad, she placed them in files with labels such as "Pending: MS Society Great Britain," or "Pending: MS Society France." Many of these letters were written by people who had seen articles about multiple sclerosis in their local newspapers, which grew out of press releases issued by the National Multiple Sclerosis Society. Although they lived in other parts of the world, they had nowhere in their own countries to turn. They wrote to the Society headquarters in New York, seeking information about the disease, and they often became members of the American organization. Sylvia knew that these individuals might someday become valuable resources when an MS organization was created in their homeland. She had the foresight to keep their correspondence on file.

Until 1948 there had been very little activity on the international front. Evelyn Opal, who had MS, had started a chapter of the U.S. Society in Montreal. When funds crossed the border, however, some of them were lost in the rate of exchange. As a result, Sylvia asked Opal to consider launching a national society in Canada, believing that the U.S. organization could not effectively undertake such a project. Opal reacted enthusiastically to the idea, and Sylvia arranged to meet with her and another Canadian with MS, Harry Bell, along with Dr. Colin Russel of Montreal, a member of the U.S. Society's Medical Advisory Board. She convinced the three Canadians that their country could support its own MS society. She gave them several boxes of MS literature, a copy of the National Society's bylaws and its chapter manual, and $25,000 in seed money that the national board had appropriated for the launch. Within months, Canada had become the second country to establish an MS society, founded with a structure similar to that of the U.S. organization. Its leadership resided in a lay board and a Medical Advisory Board, functioning side by side. The lay board had fundraising and administrative responsibilities. The Medical Advisory Board developed medical and scientific programs.

"I was so busy that I couldn't offer them much handholding," said Sylvia. "I gave them plenty of documents and literature, and wished them luck." The Canadian organization eventually evolved into a first-class operation with an excellent research program and chapters throughout the country.

Once Canada's society was up and running, Lawry's attention turned to England. She had received a letter from the United Kingdom, written by Lord Howard of Glossop. His wife had multiple sclerosis, and he had joined the National MS Society and was impressed with its activities. In his letter he invited her to come to England. He wrote, "If you can develop some interest among the scientific community here, convincing these doctors that a national society such as yours would be beneficial, I'll help get the organization off the ground."

Sylvia was excited at the prospect of spreading the movement across the Atlantic. She scheduled her first vacation in Europe, planning to spend a week in London. Before she departed, an American neurologist laughed and told her, "Things don't move that fast in the United Kingdom." But her itinerary was set and included other meetings in countries where "cures" were being reported. She arrived in London and at Lord Howard's suggestion immediately called Richard Cave, a junior clerk at the House of Lords, who helped guide her around the city. Like Lord Howard's spouse, Cave's wife had MS, and Sylvia asked him to join her for breakfast at the Hotel Savoy. Breakfast meetings were unheard of at the time in England, and in later years Cave would quip to audiences that he had wondered whether Sylvia would be dressed in a negligee when he arrived. Over breakfast in the Savoy's dining room, she showed him letters from MS families in England who had written to the Society. "An MS organization in the UK could be very important for these people, and for scientists needing support for MS research," she told him. Cave eventually became the first president of the MS society in the UK.

Later Sylvia sat down with officials at the Medical Research Council, the British counterpart to the U.S. government's National Institutes of Health. During that meeting she asked the MRC's director how much money the Council had been appropriating for MS research. He responded: "None." "Why not?" Sylvia asked. "MS is known to be a serious problem in Britain."

"We haven't received any applications for grants," he insisted. "There's just no interest in multiple sclerosis here."

"That's very strange," she told him. "Researchers in your country are turning to us for support. We're supporting research at Oxford right now. So we know about scientists who have a particular interest in MS."

In time, about one-third of the National Society's research grants were awarded to overseas investigators. The recipients were outstanding scientists—some were Nobel laureates—doing high-caliber work. In most cases, funds for MS research were not available from their own governments, and so they turned to the U.S. Society. Before her meeting at the MRC had ended, Sylvia had gained the Council's support for developing an MS society in the UK, arguing that if such an organization were established, it could stimulate scientific interest in MS and related neurological diseases.

At that point Sylvia went to National Hospital, Queens Square. Before she had departed for London, Dr. Tracy Putnam, chairman of the National Society's Medical Advisory Board, had given her the name of Dr. MacDonald Critchley, whom he said was National Hospital's chief of neurology. "He's one of the leading neurologists in England," Putnam told her, "and he'll be a good contact." When Sylvia visited Dr. Critchley in his office, he became intrigued with the idea of an MS society in the United Kingdom. He offered to host a reception on

Sylvia's last day in London and invite the UK's leading neurologists, including those from Scotland and Ireland. "It will be an opportunity for you to meet the doctors who might play a role in the medical arm of a British MS society, and hopefully we can rally their support for starting an organization here," he told her.

The day of the reception, Sylvia arrived punctually. The meeting room, however, was empty, except for Dr. Critchley and the hospital director—and a buffet table filled with food and drinks. There was no assemblage of neurologists as Sylvia had been told to expect. Thirty minutes passed. Then an hour. Finally one of the invited physicians showed up—just one. His name was Dr. Allison, and he was from Scotland. He introduced himself and told Sylvia that he had been conducting epidemiological research into MS. Then he asked about her motives for being in England.

"I'm not seeking any personal benefit, either for me or for the National MS Society in America," she told him. "My brother has MS, and I'm committed to research aimed at finding a cure for this disease. I've seen it ruin too many lives. So I'm trying to stimulate research in England, just as I've been able to do in the U.S."

Before Dr. Allison left, he told her, "I think I know why your turnout was so disappointing. You'll probably hear from me again before you leave England tomorrow."

Sylvia returned to her hotel room, feeling despondent. The dismal turnout had really disappointed her. Although she didn't know it at the time, medical egos and internal politics had spoiled the event. Dr. Douglas McAlpine, a prominent figure in the British neurological community, considered himself to be England's foremost MS authority. He had written the most comprehensive textbook about multiple sclerosis to date, and he was upset that Sylvia had first approached Dr. Critchley and not him. He had become suspicious of her reasons for visiting the UK, and in the hours before the reception he had apparently contacted his colleagues and urged them to ignore the event—which nearly everyone did.

Sylvia's hopes had been high when she came to England, but without winning the support of the neurological community she felt as though her trip was wasted. But while packing her suitcase and preparing to depart England the following day, the phone in her room rang. It was Dr. Allison. "Before you leave town," he said, "you must go to Middlesex Hospital to meet with Dr. McAlpine. He'd like to see you at nine o'clock tomorrow."

The next morning Sylvia took a cab to the hospital. Dr. McAlpine, adorned in his white coat, met her at the entrance. He ushered her into his office and almost immediately opened his file drawers. "Here are the records of more than a thousand multiple sclerosis patients whom I've treated," he said. "No one in the UK cares for more MS patients than I." Then he asked why she had contacted Dr. Critchley rather than him, and listened while she explained that she had only followed the advice of Dr. Putnam. By the end of their meeting, McAlpine sensed her sincerity and offered the encouragement she had wanted to hear. "I'll support your efforts," he said, "and you'll have a proper medical advisory board for a British Society."

The MS Society of Great Britain and Northern Ireland was formally created in 1953 with Dr. McAlpine as the chairman of its Medical Advisory Board. At the first meeting of the new society in London, a line of people with an interest in MS stretched around the block, waiting to get in. They were desperate for hope and information.

From England, Sylvia traveled to France and met with

Pierre Hansel, who had MS and used a wheelchair. He had expressed interest in establishing a national organization in France. Hansel lived in the countryside, about twenty miles from Paris, and on a bumpy cab ride to his home, Sylvia became ill. "I succumbed completely to the lobster I had eaten the night before," she said. Doing her best to remain composed in spite of her discomfort, she discussed the elements necessary to create a national society and urged Hansel to find people to help him get the organization started—and then she quickly departed.

Sylvia traveled on to Vienna. Before she left the United States she had heard rumors about a so-called cure for MS that was being administered in Austria. She arranged a meeting with the doctor who had been promoting the therapy, hoping that he really had developed a breakthrough. In fact she learned that it had been an erroneous report and that the neurologist himself was furious that his own research had been distorted by rumormongers.

Although disappointed, she spent a few days in Austria stimulating interest in starting an MS society there. The same thing happened in Belgium. Before long, national societies were formally launched in one country after another, with Germany leading the way, followed by Austria, Denmark, Sweden, Belgium, Switzerland, South Africa, Ireland, the Netherlands, and Norway. When Sylvia returned exhausted from her "vacation" in Europe, Edward Bernays asked, "What do you think of people abroad?" Knowing that Bernays was a nephew of Sigmund Freud, Sylvia assumed that he was expecting a complex, psychologically oriented response. But she said simply, "I found that if you can reach them, they're basically no different than us. They encounter the same problems in coping with MS as we do, and they react in the same way." Then she added, "My most effective tool for reaching out to them was a broad smile. It overcame every language barrier. Nothing warmed these people up as quickly as a smile."

From that point Sylvia continued trying to stimulate the growth of the MS movement internationally. Still, one woman could do only so much. When a neurologist in Argentina repeatedly asked for her help in establishing a national society in that country, she politely declined invitations to travel there, simply because she couldn't schedule them into her overloaded calendar. "When I'd receive requests like these, I became convinced that it was time for a coordinated global effort to conquer multiple sclerosis, led by a full-time professional organizer," she said.

That was the next step.

21

WITH MEMBERSHIPS of national MS societies growing, Sylvia Lawry began to ponder the feasibility of establishing an international federation. Her hope was that such an organization would help generate international scientific interest in MS research. It could sponsor an annual conference where member societies might share information about research programs in their own countries, and about treatment practices that could improve the quality of life of persons with the disease. The conference could also host workshops on services, fundraising, and public relations. The federation might promote the establishment of new MS societies in nations where none presently existed, and disseminate educational information about the disease and its management. So in the early 1960s, Sylvia researched the ways in which the international movement in other voluntary health organizations—including those dedicated to conquering cancer and tuberculosis—had evolved. With her energies already spread much too thin, however, she convinced the national board to form a committee, called the International Programs Committee and headed by

Charles Meares, to study the feasibility and role of an international MS federation.

When Sylvia learned about an international rehabilitation conference scheduled in Copenhagen, she decided to gather representatives of fourteen national societies there to discuss the feasibility of a global organization. She asked Lizzie Almond, a social worker who was executive director of the Danish society, to find a room for the meeting and enter it into the conference program.

Sylvia anticipated a giant leap in the international movement—until she arrived for the meeting. It was a déjà vu experience, reminiscent of that earlier gathering in London where the UK's leading neurologists were no-shows. Not even Lizzie Almond was in sight. "I found out that Lizzie had been fired by Dr. Torbin Fog, president of the Danish MS society, after he discovered that she, a lay person, had made these arrangements for a meeting involving lay people rather than physicians without consulting him," Sylvia reported. "He was absolutely livid, and had our meeting removed from the conference program. As far as he was concerned, there wasn't going to be a meeting or an international federation."

Later Sylvia learned that Dr. Fog had consulted with other European physicians, and they all believed that the United States was staging an "invasion" designed to take control of the worldwide MS movement. He was also upset that lay people were encroaching on an area that, in Europe, had traditionally been reserved solely for physicians and scientists. At that time, no European health agency was being run by lay volunteers, and Dr. Fog and his fellow doctors were not eager to relinquish any of their control.

With no sign of a meeting room in Copenhagen, Sylvia felt both angry and frantic. She began trying to track down the people whom she had invited to her meeting: Kathe Wilbrand from Germany, Ingegerd Bursie from Sweden, Dr. Brian Pringle from Ireland, and representatives from England, Norway, and other countries. One by one she contacted all of them, finding some of them wandering the hallways of the conference center, looking for her. She quickly changed her hotel room to a suite and asked everyone to gather there that evening.

"It turned out to be a magnificent meeting," said Sylvia. "We discussed strategy, and whether there would be support for an international MS society. There was so much excitement in the room that the meeting lasted well into the night—until two in the morning." A consensus was forming for the establishment of a global organization.

Dr. Pringle, who had organized the MS society in Ireland, was the only physician at the meeting. He had been President of the Royal Academy of Medicine of Ireland and thus was an influential force in his country's medical community. In later years both he and Sylvia told stories of how she often woke him with middle-of-the-night phone calls from the United States, thanks to her frequent miscalculations of the time difference between New York and Dublin. "He never told me that I had awakened him," Sylvia said. "I guess he didn't want to embarrass me, so he would just handle the problem or answer my questions, and then go back to sleep."

At the end of that formal gathering in Sylvia's suite, the group made plans to assemble again. They decided that the next meeting would be held in Vienna and that representatives from throughout the world would be invited to consider formally creating an international organization. Sylvia was given the responsibility of developing bylaws for the new federation.

Meanwhile Dr. Fog and Dr. Henk Dassel of the Netherlands, a renowned figure in rehabilitation medicine in Europe, called a meeting of their own, bringing together representatives from the existing European societies to talk about forming a European federation that would exclude participation by the United States and other non-European national societies. "Why do we need an international organization?" Dr. Fog asked the group. "Let's have a European federation of MS societies and not risk domination by the United States."

With this potential rebellion among the European physicians, Sylvia felt she needed a trump card that would make it harder for anyone to veto a global federation. She decided to take a bold step: she proposed to the National MS Society board that it provide a seed-money grant of $100,000 to establish the international organization. "If start-up funding is available," she told the board, "there is greater likelihood of winning worldwide support." Board sentiment generally favored her recommendation, but there were reservations.

Board member John F. McGillicuddy, a supporter of the global movement, recalled, "I felt strongly that we had to try to make this an international effort rather than only an American one. I believed that the benefit over the long term would more than justify the relatively modest outlays that would be necessary to get the federation up and running. However, those who opposed it thought it would siphon off money and resources that we could use here."

When a vote was taken, the national board recognized the potential value of an international coalition of societies and approved the $100,000 grant. Board members agreed with Sylvia that an international federation could engage a broad array of scientists around the world to study MS.

To win over remaining skeptics in the United States, Sylvia pointed out that a large number of the recent winners of the

Nobel Prize for Medicine had been from outside the country. "None of us really cares where the cure or effective treatments come from," she said. "We just want that cure to happen. An international organization is one way to stimulate research abroad that can help MS patients everywhere."

In 1965 a formal organizational meeting was scheduled in Vienna. "We invited all interested parties to attend, including Dr. Fog and his allies," said Sylvia. "I realized that we would need to win their support for an international federation to be effective. Toward that end, I would need to convince Dr. Fog that there was interest in the federation on continents other than Europe, and that this wasn't some kind of sinister American plot."

To prepare for the meeting, Lawry called upon Ingegerd Bursie for help. Bursie, whose daughter had MS, had founded the Swedish MS society. She was well known throughout Europe, thanks in part to her husband's service as Swedish ambassador to a number of countries. Bursie had met Sylvia when the two women happened to sit next to each other at a neurological conference. When the Vienna meeting was scheduled, Bursie agreed to travel from one country to another, personally urging the leadership of the existing societies to send representatives to the meeting. At the same time Dr. James Q. Simmons, Jr., the National Society's Director of Medical Programs and a former army officer, used his military connections to travel throughout Europe, meeting with key neurologists to gain support for an international federation.

Meanwhile Dr. Fog was devising a counterstrategy. He still hoped to form a Europe-only organization, and he continued to rally support among neurologists on the continent as well as lay leaders of the European MS societies, gaining commitments from a growing number of them. At the same time, however,

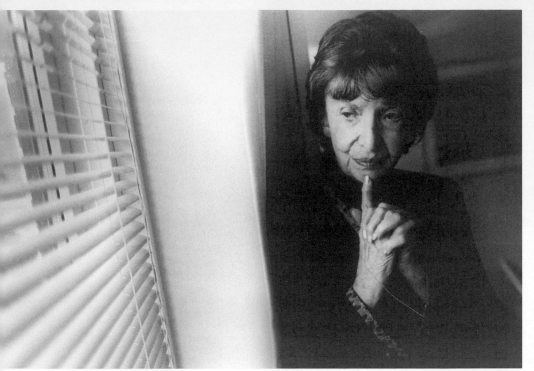

Sylvia Lawry, founder-director of the National Multiple Sclerosis Society and the Multiple Sclerosis International Federation.

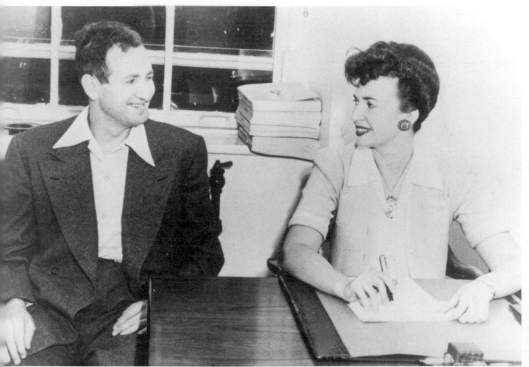

Sylvia with her brother Bernard, who inspired her to confront MS, in the Society's first office at the New York Academy of Medicine in the late 1940s.

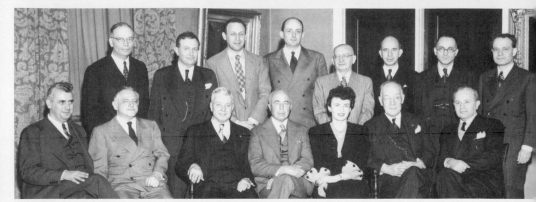

The first Medical Advisory Board of the National MS Society, 1946.

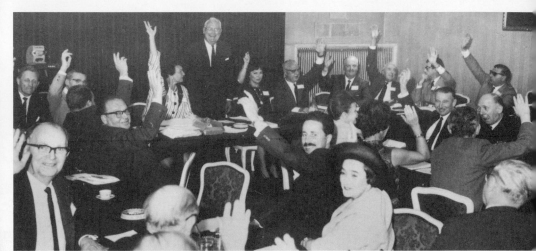

The International Federation of MS Societies, precursor of the Multiple Sclerosis International Federation, ratifies its original charter, 1967.

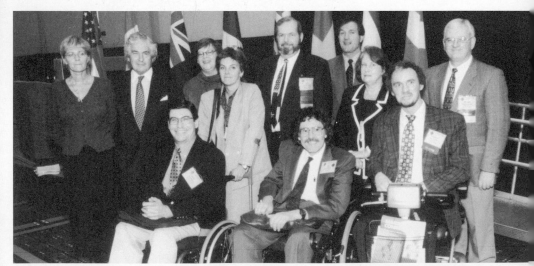

Delegates to the International Leadership Conference in Atlanta, 1996.

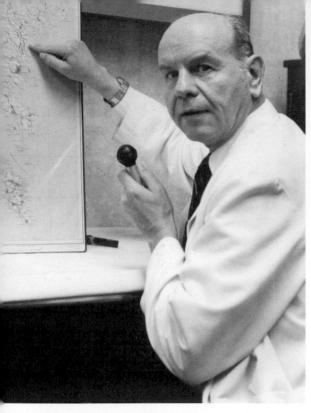

MS researcher Dr. John F. Kurtzke.

r. Elvin Kabat, who received the very first grant for MS research from the Society for the
dvancement of Multiple Sclerosis Research, precursor of the National Multiple Sclerosis
ociety.   [Rene Perez]

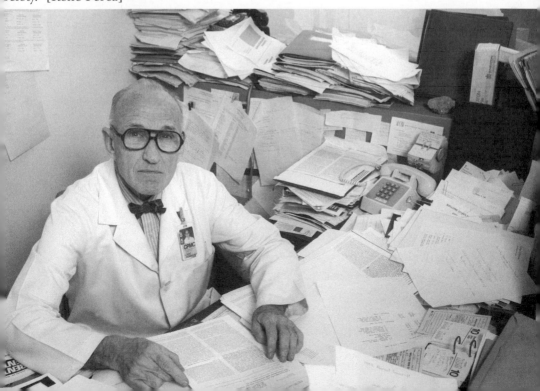

MS researchers at work ...

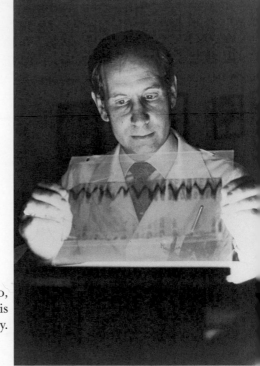

Dr. Raymond P. Roos, University of Chicago, studying a gel run in his laboratory.

James Connor, Ph.D., MS researcher at Hershey Medical Center in Pennsylvania.

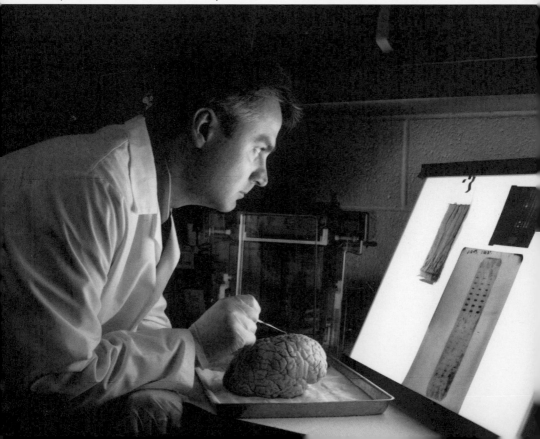

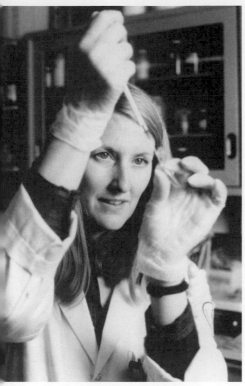

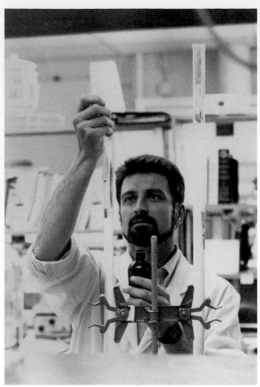

. Janet Lee, researcher in molecular
munobiology at Memorial Sloan-
ttering Cancer Center, New York.

Dr. Oscar Bizzezero, School of Medicine,
University of New Mexico.

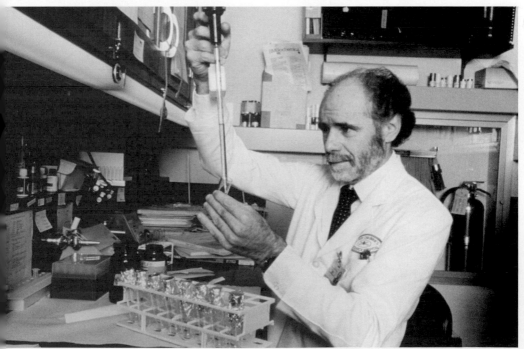

. G. G. Re transferring a virus culture at St. Jude Hospital, Memphis, Tennessee.

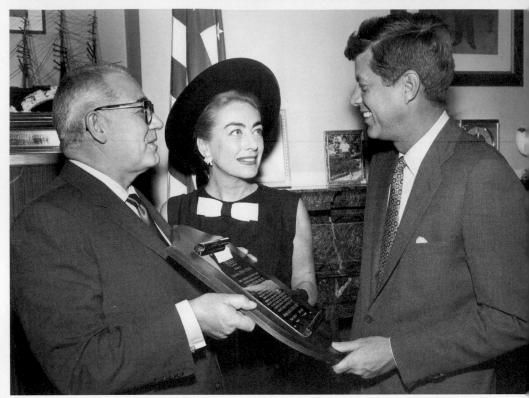

Alfred N. Steele, who died suddenly on the eve of the 1959 MS Hope Chest campaign, presents a plaque to former national MS Hope Chest chairman, Senator John F. Kennec Joan Crawford, Mrs. Steele (center), took over as campaign chairman following her husband's death.

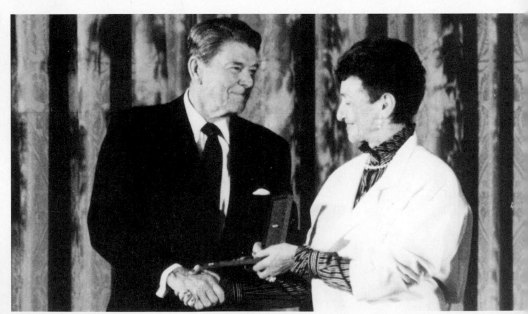

President Ronald Reagan presents Sylvia Lawry with the President's Volunteer Action Award at the White House, 1987.

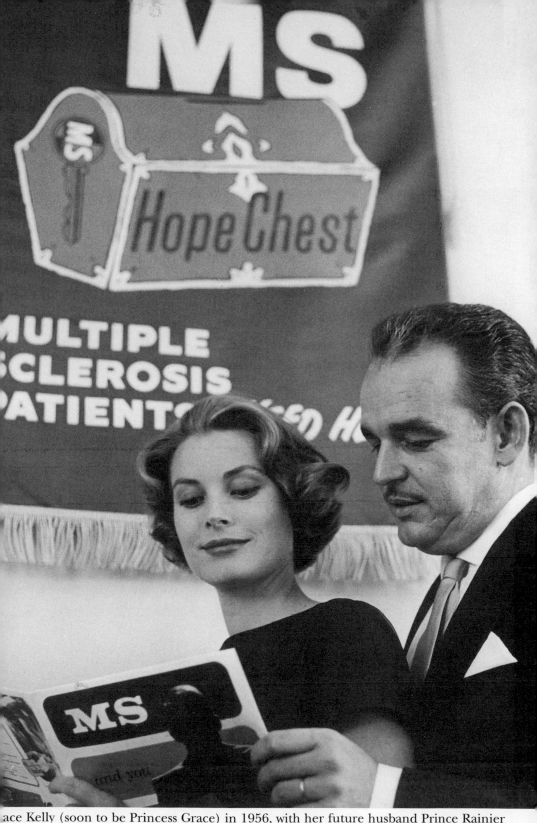

ace Kelly (soon to be Princess Grace) in 1956, with her future husband Prince Rainier Monaco—she chaired the MS Society's Women's Activities before her marriage.

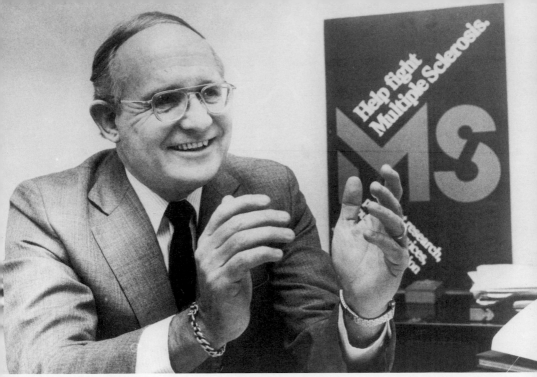

Admiral Thor Hanson,
president and CEO of the
National MS Society,
1982–1992.

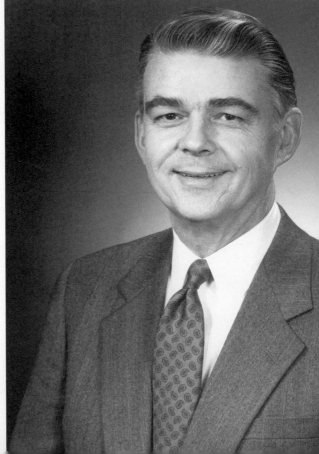

General Mike Dugan, current
president and CEO of the
National MS Society.

Chapter 21

Sylvia was calling or writing to her international contacts, appealing for their backing. She placed a call to Dr. Geoffrey Dean, who was conducting MS studies in South Africa. He had discovered that among eleven million Bantu natives there wasn't a single case of MS. Dr. Dean agreed to fly to Vienna for the meeting to explain to the assemblage that interest in the international movement existed in his part of the world. In fact, he said, there was an MS society in South Africa that wished to be part of the global network. Sylvia also contacted A. M. Wilson, an Australian airline executive who had MS and who promised to sing the praises of the international federation in Vienna and insist that his country be included.

Finally, Sylvia pulled out the ace up her sleeve. She convinced Shirley Temple Black, a member of the national board, to join the American delegation to the meeting. In September 1965, Black traveled with Sylvia, William Breed, Jr., Charles Meares, and Dr. Houston Merritt to Austria to try to persuade the other delegates, including some of the world's most respected neurologists, that an international organization deserved a chance.

As the meeting in Vienna approached, tensions were high. Within the worldwide neurological community and among nonphysicians invited to the event, opinions were strongly divided. Fifty representatives from fifteen countries attended the session at the Palais Palffy, and no one was certain what the ultimate outcome would be. When William Breed gaveled the meeting to order, almost immediately it became a highly charged event. Sylvia announced that the board of the National MS Society in the United States had approved a $100,000 start-up grant. "This will relieve all member societies of any financial burden for the next two years," she said. She hoped that this announcement would allay the reluctance of some delegates.

But not everyone was convinced. Representatives from each country—including several that hadn't yet formally created a national society—described their concerns over America's control of the federation. Finally, just moments before a vote was to be taken, Shirley Temple Black rose to her feet. She looked around the room, making eye contact with many of the delegates. Then she asked, "What have you got to lose?" There really was no risk, she argued, financial or otherwise. "We're all here for the same reason," she insisted, "and that's to wipe out multiple sclerosis." Again she posed the question, "What have you got to lose?"

The room became silent. Almost instantly the anti-federation sentiment melted. Breed called for the casting of ballots. The result: a unanimous vote in favor of the global organization. Even Dr. Fog and his allies joined the consensus. Before long he became one of the International Federation's most enthusiastic and productive supporters, as did Dr. Dassel.

The Vienna delegates collectively signed a certificate of intent to create the federation. They also planned to meet again in London once a committee had drawn up a proposed constitution and bylaws for the new group. "We really shouldn't underestimate the credit that Shirley Temple Black deserves in this," said Meares. "All of these brilliant, grey-bearded scientists wanted to meet Shirley. They remembered her from when she was a little kid in the movies, and she still had plenty of appeal. They were nearly tripping over one another to have their photograph taken with her. It was really something. She was very helpful."

The American delegation returned home feeling triumphant. When the National MS Society held its Twentieth Anniversary Conference in Washington, D.C., in 1966, the attendees celebrated not only a hallmark event in the Society's own history but also the dawning of the global federation. By then, thanks to the energy and dedication of the National Society's staff and volunteers, the American organization's growth had also been dramatic. In 1966, for the first time, the Society budgeted $1 million for research to be expended the following calendar year. It was an impressive record of humanitarian accomplishment.

At the Twentieth Anniversary Conference, the four hundred delegates included representatives from twelve national societies from other countries. William Breed spoke dramatically before a hushed audience as he held up the signed certificate of intent from the Vienna meeting and read portions of it: "We the undersigned do hereby agree that there will be organized an International Federation of Multiple Sclerosis Societies. That such a Federation has as its purposes to coordinate and further the work of national multiple sclerosis organizations throughout the world; to stimulate and encourage scientific research respecting multiple sclerosis and related neurological diseases; to aid individuals who are in any way disabled as a result of multiple sclerosis and related diseases; to collect and disseminate scientific and educational information relating to multiple sclerosis; and to provide counsel and active help in the further development of voluntary national multiple sclerosis organizations or concerning the formation of such organizations."

Breed set the document down, looked up at the crowd, and concluded, "These are the purposes of the Federation. They are broad and imaginative in scope. However excellent our aims may be, the true strength lies within our relationships. Unanimity of purpose was sought and achieved. We are now one body, cohesive in spirit and objectives. We are a family of nations aroused and eager to work together for our common purpose—to fight multiple sclerosis throughout the world."

The delegates gave Breed a standing ovation.

In 1967, attention turned to the House of Lords, one of England's most august bodies, composed of bishops, princes, and other nobles. Its chamber in Parliament is decorated with elegantly carved thrones and is an impressive setting that has traditionally been off limits for anything other than parliamentary business. Thanks to Lord Howard and Richard Cave, however, the final organizational meeting of the International Federation convened in the House of Lords in August, presided over by Cave. It was the first time in history that the House of Lords had been made available to an outside group. The delegates gathered in the Moses Room and thrashed out, fine-tuned, and voted on the constitution and bylaws. They reached a final agreement and passed the document around the room for signatures.

"On the rear wall behind Richard Cave there was a large oil painting of Moses handing down the Ten Commandments," said Sylvia. Nathan Mobley, a U.S. delegate to that meeting, a member of the Board of Directors of the National MS Society, and vice president of the Chubb Group of Insurance Companies, said, "Here we are, formulating the Ten Commandments of the worldwide MS movement."

Sylvia noted, "That parallel was scintillating. All of us had a sense that something historic was happening."

The new organization was formally given the name International Federation of Multiple Sclerosis Societies (IFMSS). It consisted of seventeen member societies. William Breed was selected honorary chairman. Sylvia Lawry was designated as secretary. Shirley Temple Black was named international chairwoman of volunteers. Dr. H. Houston Merritt was assigned the task of organizing an International Medical Advisory Board. Two months later, John Horner was elected the first permanent secretary-general of the Federation, with the secretariat based in Austria. The city of Vienna had agreed to subsidize the operating costs of the new organization's headquarters. Other attendees at the meeting were prominent figures in the MS movement, including Dr. Brian Pringle of Ireland, Ingegerd Bursie of Sweden, Edith Bors of Norway, and Kathe Wilbrand of Germany.

It was a memorable moment in the MS movement—an organized global assault on the disease. Nevertheless, even with the dawning of the IFMSS, there remained isolated grumbling over whether such an organization was really necessary. In the United States, sentiment at the National MS Society's headquarters generally supported the global effort, recognizing the crucial role it could play in stimulating research internationally. In other parts of the world, however, some MS leaders were so preoccupied with their own national societies, and felt so much pressure to meet the immediate needs in their respective countries, that the international movement ranked low on their priority list. "There were doubting Thomases who should have been behind this, but weren't," said Sylvia. "Of course, I recognized that they needed to pay attention to the task of building their own national organizations. But some of them, I believe, were simply unable to grasp what could lie ahead if some of their energies were directed at supporting the International Federation.

"I tend to be the eternal optimist, so I didn't foresee some of the problems that arose," Sylvia added. "Frankly, I was always shocked over any resistance to the Federation."

The global movement grew steadily. "I believe that my

greatest value to the international movement has been my ability to recruit and motivate people," Sylvia observed. "Individuals from around the world with an interest in MS, when they've been in New York on business or holidays, have come to meet with me at the National Society's offices to discuss the issues and the problems they're facing. Many of them have left feeling more focused on what needed to be done when they returned home."

As with the National MS Society, the people behind the International Federation became its greatest asset. F. C. ("Bud") Wiser, Jr., the first president of the International Federation, was also the president of Trans World Airlines. When he traveled the world on business, he dealt with Federation matters on the same trips. He also recruited TWA's advertising agency—Wells Rich Greene—to represent the Society pro bono. Later, J. Walter Thompson took over the advertising campaigns and worked without charge.

Dr. Hans Hoff evolved into an influential force on the Federation's Medical Advisory Board. While on staff of the New York Neurological Institute, Hoff had received a grant from the U.S. Society to travel abroad to study the status of multiple sclerosis throughout the world. Because of this international perspective, he had the background to provide crucial input for the scientific arm of the new global organization. He moved to Vienna, where he ultimately became the father of neurology in Austria.

By 1969, when the first quadrennial meeting of the IFMSS council was held in New York, the Federation was functioning with great expectations. At that gathering the organization presented its first Jean-Martin Charcot Award, named after the pioneering scientist who had first characterized MS in detail a hundred years earlier. The prize was created to honor a scientist who had made a significant contribution in the field of MS research. Ironically, that award was given to Dr. Douglas McAlpine, the British neurologist who had once resisted Sylvia Lawry's organizational efforts in the UK.

The early years of the Federation were fraught with continuing suspicions. At home, although support for the IFMSS remained strong, some skeptics feared that other countries would lean on the National MS Society as the primary source of funding for the international organization. "Overseas we continued to fight the feeling that anything we proposed was a sign that Americans were trying to dominate the organization," Sylvia recalled. "It took about five years to allay those concerns and convince the member nations that we had nothing to gain except the progress being made against multiple sclerosis."

As the years passed, Sylvia and other leaders of the international movement were warmly embraced. At one memorable International Federation reception at the Royal Palace in Belgium, Queen Fabiola greeted the MS organization's twenty-person executive committee delegation. She was dressed unpretentiously and made the group feel welcome. As tea was served, the guests and Queen Fabiola sat in a circle, and the queen asked everyone to describe how they had become involved in the MS movement. When the queen's turn came, she said simply, "I'm interested in MS because someone in whom I'm interested has it. Thanks to all of you for everything you're doing." Before the delegation departed, they posed for a photograph with Queen Fabiola. Sylvia positioned herself in the back row as the photographer prepared for a few shots. But when the queen noticed Sylvia's location, she would have none of it. She got up from her front-row seat, took Sylvia by the hand, and insisted that she sit next to her in the front.

"When we departed, the queen accompanied us out to the

driveway, made sure we were seated comfortably in our cars, and waved goodbye," said Sylvia. "Despite her royal status, she couldn't have been more down to earth."

Sylvia never wavered in her determination to attract prominent people who were in a position to assist the Federation and its member societies worldwide, convincing them to join the leadership ranks of the global movement. "After these individuals attended our international conferences and met young people with multiple sclerosis—some of whom were in wheelchairs, in their teens and twenties—the pathos of it reached them, and they became involved," said Sylvia. "And the campaign slogan we had used in the U.S.—'Someone you know has MS'—touched people abroad as well. Many people would say to me, 'Yes, I do know someone with MS.'"

In those early years when Sylvia was trying to persuade William Breed, Jr., that the establishment of the Federation made sense, she offered her most persuasive arguments, then quipped, "It's going to make my job a lot easier, because I won't have to spend my vacations in Europe, trying on my own to keep the movement going."

Breed laughed and replied prophetically, "Believe me, it's going to make your job harder!"

And that was so. "Mr. Breed was right," she said. "It was like having two full-time jobs."

22

I N THE 1960s, few corporate executives were more respected than Daniel J. Haughton. He was board chairman of the Lockheed Aircraft Corporation and keenly understood the workings of American industry. He also had intimate knowledge of multiple sclerosis because his wife, Jean, had MS. The disease was as much a part of his day-to-day life as making multimillion-dollar decisions in the Lockheed boardroom.

Haughton was probably one of the busiest men in the country, but that didn't stop Sylvia Lawry from approaching him to take on the challenge of the presidency of the National Multiple Sclerosis Society. He had earned money to attend college by working in the mines digging coal. Years later, as a corporate executive, he earned a reputation as a skilled volunteer fundraiser. Sylvia believed that, more than anyone else, he was capable of leading the Society toward its ultimate goal. She became so convinced that his presence was crucial to the Society's future that, when she met with him, she said, "I want to make it clear that if you become our president, you have no obligation to keep me as executive director. You should feel free to make your own choice of a person in whom you have complete confidence."

Once Haughton had served a brief period as a member of the national board and had gotten to know Sylvia better, he told her, "The *only* basis on which I'd take the presidency would be if you'd continue as executive director." In fact Haughton agreed to assume the presidency of the Society in 1969, and he held that title until 1973; thereafter he became board chairman for another three years.

Haughton's self-assurance and take-charge approach raised enthusiasm levels among the troops at both the national headquarters and chapter offices. Despite his stature in corporate America, he was unpretentious and approachable (a newspaper article described him as "the Will Rogers of industry"). His warmth and gregariousness were magnetic, and his colorful Southern charm captivated everyone who met him in the MS world. Haughton himself once told an MS national leadership conference, "Go after the top leaders in your community to become involved in your chapters. Just go meet these people. They're no different than anyone else." For the individuals who met Haughton through the National MS Society, he never put on airs. He expected everyone to give at least 100 percent, nothing less, and never lose focus on getting the better of MS.

John McGillicuddy, who was president of Manufacturers Hanover Trust Company when Haughton recruited him for the National Society board, said that he had initially believed that the Lockheed president and Sylvia Lawry would often clash. "They were both very demanding, hard-charging people, and at times they did indeed have their differences," he said. "But Sylvia never had anything other than tremendous admiration for Dan and what he had accomplished, and she loved the fact that he wanted to get things done immediately, because that was her feeling as well. In the same way, Dan thought the world of Sylvia because of her dedication to the Society."

National board member L. Palmer Brown made similar observations. "There was no more dedicated person than Dan, nor a more ambitious and capable one. He came in like a hawk, and said, 'We're going to expand this Society and get it supporting the research that needs to be done.' He recruited top-notch business people to serve on the national board. He went from city to city, talking to chapter members. He personally solicited funds all over the United States, and because of his stature at Lockheed he was able to get in virtually every door. He was a master of persuasion and convinced Sylvia Lawry to do things organizationally that she would not have done otherwise. He really breathed new life into the Society."

According to Brown, Haughton insisted that Sylvia broaden her vision and no longer feel the need to read every letter that went out of the office. "Sylvia was so dedicated that she wanted to be sure everything was right," said Brown. "But the workload became so overwhelming that there just wasn't time to do that anymore."

Longtime Society leaders like Brown considered Haughton to be a pivotal figure in the history of the organization. "In 1978, when I was elected chairman of the National MS Society, our total gross income was about $15 million, and when I left the position it was $25 million," said Brown. "I believe that growth was due not to my own activities but to the groundwork that Dan Haughton had laid. His efforts catapulted the Society into a period of growth by leaps and bounds."

Shortly after Sylvia convinced Haughton to assume the presidency of the Society, she received a phone call from an executive with the American Red Cross in California, who headed one of its divisions. He congratulated her on lassoing the Lockheed chief. Haughton was on the national board of the Red Cross and had been volunteer chairman of a record-breaking Red Cross fundraising campaign in California. Sometime later, his affiliation with that organization also led Sylvia to suggest a project that, with the help of Mary Goodyear, a member of both boards, was launched jointly by the National MS Society and the American Red Cross to care for persons with MS at home.

The Red Cross's excellent facilities for training, transportation, and education led to a major upgrading of services for persons with MS. "You've got the world's greatest volunteer fundraiser," the caller from California told Sylvia. That observation couldn't have been more accurate. In 1969 the new Society president announced a plan—the so-called Haughton Plan—which called for raising $10 million in five years specifically for an aggressively expanded MS research program. The $10 million goal was double the amount allocated for research by the Society during the previous five-year period; half would be raised by chapter volunteers, and the other half would be solicited by a special national development committee whose members would approach corporations and foundations in twenty-six major cities.

In an interview, Haughton promised that every dollar raised by the special national committee would be spent on research. "There will be no deductions for fundraising, promotion, public relations or administrative expenses; every gift will be placed in a special research fund account and used in its entirety to make payments to universities, medical schools, or hospitals for approved research programs." It became the most intense fundraising campaign since the Society's establishment. Not surprisingly, it was successful. Haughton's goals were reached and even exceeded.

Whenever Haughton met with Sylvia at the National MS Society's office in New York, he asked for a cup of coffee and then put twenty-five cents down on the desk in front of her. Sylvia recalls, "His message was, 'Don't spend the Society's money on things like coffee; there are much more important ways to allocate our funds.'"

Even as the Society, under Haughton's guidance, thrived, MS remained unbroken. Its cause remained unknown. The disease process was poorly understood. Effective treatments were desperately needed. In studies of animals and human brain tissue cultures, investigators sought evidence of why and how one person with MS might recover from an attack while another individual's disability increased with each episode. The ultimate hope, according to one scientist, was to discover a means of influencing the cells and controlling their future so that MS could be controlled as well.

One line of aggressive research in the 1960s sought to discover if a common virus might be a triggering agent for MS. The virus, theorized some scientists, might cause seemingly trivial damage in the central nervous system that could liberate a tiny component of its fat and protein material. This substance might act like a foreign agent and set into motion an autoimmune response. The viral infection, the scientists believed, might not be the root cause of MS but perhaps triggers the autoimmune mechanism.

Meanwhile, Dan Haughton insisted upon an expansion of services to people with MS and of public education programs. In 1969 he announced, "The Medical Programs Department hopes to stimulate more than two hundred MS clinics, within the ability of each community to provide initial funding. This department will also employ a staff member to seek locations for such clinics where medical school and government agency cooperation can be assured. We will also attempt to develop and charter new chapters until the Society reaches into every county of this nation."

Haughton's vision for the Society was ambitious and un-wavering. "I'll tell you this about Dan," said John McGillicuddy. "No one was more committed to this cause than he was. Because his wife had multiple sclerosis, he felt very strongly about the need to find a cure. So he approached his presidency with a 'take-no-prisoners' attitude, and what you could get done to-morrow, you might as well get done today. He exerted a lot of pressure on the staff to achieve, and I think that was important because we were still a relatively small organization."

As busy as Haughton remained with his responsibilities at Lockheed, he was always available when needed for Society business, never missing a single board meeting. At every op-portunity he helped give the Society greater public visibility. When he visited the White House, in an Oval Office ceremony he presented President Richard Nixon with a special MS Hope Chest Award. Upon Haughton's death, his will left $450,000 to the National Society.

23

WHEN THE WORLD REJOICED at the development of the polio vaccine, most of the credit was deservedly given to Dr. Jonas Salk. Few people knew about the contribution of Dr. Harry Weaver.

Dr. Weaver was a neurophysiologist and had been a professor of anatomy at Wayne State University College of Medicine in Detroit. In 1946 he moved to New York to become the director of research at the National Foundation for Infantile Paralysis, and until 1953 he was the master architect of the polio research program. He was largely responsible for getting Dr. Salk interested in polio research. Just before the creation of the National MS Society in 1946, when Sylvia Lawry was trying to convince the National Foundation to incorporate MS into its mission, Weaver was one of the few voices there who favored that move. As part of the campaign against polio, he encouraged basic research, though he demanded that it hold the promise of contributing to the ultimate solution to the crippling disease. He had a knack for recruiting scientists who would pursue avenues of research that he believed would bring the Foundation another step closer to relegating polio to the history books. He became so strongly committed to the cause that when Salk needed subjects to receive the vaccine in early trials, both Weaver and his son volunteered to be inoculated.

Dr. Thomas Rivers, the Rockefeller Institute virologist who served on the National MS Society's Medical Advisory Board, once described Dr. Weaver as having "a wonderful quality of being bold. In research you often need a person like Harry Weaver around, someone to encourage people to see what the grass is like on the other side. In other words, a catalyst. Harry Weaver performed that function beautifully."

In 1966, after millions of children had received the Salk vaccine, the National Multiple Sclerosis Society began looking for someone to assume the reins of the organization's research program. The national board did not want a research director who would simply lean back and wait for grant applications to come in. Instead it sought a director who would step out and stir things up, actively stimulating interest in multiple sclerosis. It wanted someone who would play an aggressive role in pushing the science of MS forward.

The Medical Advisory Board appointed a search committee, headed by Dr. H. Houston Merritt, to find a leading scientist to fill the job. Merritt had worked with Weaver in the polio program, and nearly every candidate who was put forward for the job with the National MS Society drew the following reaction from Merritt: "He's no Harry Weaver."

As the selection process dragged on, Sylvia sat down at her typewriter and wrote a letter to Dr. Weaver. At the end of it, she wrote, "I have an abiding interest in meeting you so I can see what I'm supposed to be looking for."

Not long after receiving this letter, Weaver agreed to come to New York to confer with her. He was enjoying retirement in

San Clemente, California, living in a beautiful home overlooking the Pacific. During their lengthy meeting, Sylvia explained the desperate need to find a cure for MS. She drew parallels between the crippling nature of polio and MS. Then, as the meeting ended, she asked him to consider becoming the director of all of the Society's research programs.

"You can work from San Clemente," she told him. "But you will be traveling a lot. We also need you in New York for our Medical Advisory Board meetings and our Peer Review Committee meetings." It didn't take him long to make up his mind. His wife urged him to take the new position, and he agreed. "Count me in!" he said. "When would I start?"

Overnight, morale at the Society soared. "After all, Harry Weaver was the man who had played a critical role in developing the polio vaccine," said Sylvia. "In the scientific community, the message was, 'If Weaver is taking on MS, it must be a hot subject.'" In a dramatic moment in 1969, Dr. Jonas Salk appeared before the National Society's board and said, "The greatest thing that could have happened to MS was to recruit Weaver as your research director." He added, "If the truth were told, Weaver advised me on what needed to be done at every stage of the development of the polio vaccine." As Dr. Salk closed his remarks, he said with conviction, "Every disease has its time. The time has arrived to find the answer to MS."

Weaver was a great proselytizer, as Sylvia had hoped. He began aggressively encouraging scientists to take on the National Society's mission as their own. Even so, at his first Board of Directors meeting, when he was asked if he could project what his research plans would be, he said, "I won't make any predictions at this time. Ask me that question a year from now. I need to know a great deal more than I do now about what is already taking place in the research labs. I intend to visit every laboratory in the world working on MS, and after that I will submit my plan."

In the next twelve months Weaver visited dozens of labs and met with scores of scientists. Then he presented the board with a five-year research program, wrapped in plenty of hope. When he spoke at an MS seminar for medical writers in Washington, D.C., he opened with these words: "We've been on a research plateau for a long time now. But new facts, some isolated just now, indicate we are entering into a period of rapid progress."

Several of the other scientists who spoke at that symposium proclaimed that MS might reflect a breakdown in the body's immune system. Dr. John Sever, a government researcher, suggested that MS might be the legacy of a childhood infection. Dr. Rune Stjernholm of Western Reserve University School of Medicine in Cleveland described his efforts to develop a blood test for diagnosing MS. His research, he explained, indicated that certain white blood cells are altered structurally and metabolically in people with MS—a marker that might evolve into a diagnostic tool.

Buoyed by Dr. Weaver's high expectations, Society president Daniel Haughton felt even more strongly motivated to raise the money that his research director needed. In the aftermath of his meetings with many scientists, Haughton singled out three areas in particular in which research funding should be channeled:

An investigation of the abnormal immune response suspected in MS.

The possibility that multiple sclerosis was an infectious process, and that a slow-acting virus was responsible for MS.

Studies on whether a drug called cyclophosphamide, which had arrested the progress of paralysis in animals with an

MS-like disease, might be useful in humans with multiple sclerosis.

Before the 1960s ended, the first successful controlled clinical trial of an MS treatment was completed. Patients with MS exacerbations had been given the steroid ACTH intramuscularly, and in a carefully designed study their response was compared to a group receiving a placebo. This research demonstrated that ACTH was superior to placebo, accelerating the recovery from acute MS episodes. The study also established placebo-controlled, double-blind clinical trials as the gold standard for studies of new MS therapies, a standard which has lasted into the twenty-first century.

In 1969, as a new decade and a renewed sense of optimism were about to dawn, the National MS Society Annual Report reflected Daniel Haughton's impatience. He wrote: "President Franklin D. Roosevelt once said how, following his attack of polio, he had spent a year learning to wiggle his big toe. It is in this perspective that I report on the results of the initial year of the Research Development Fund appeal.

"I am not content that we made a good beginning. We did learn how to wiggle our big toe. I am discontented with the pace of progress in raising the funds, measured against the explosively expanding leads about multiple sclerosis emerging from the laboratories, leads which must be pursued without undue delay."

24

THE 1970s were years when developments in other areas of medicine, such as genetic engineering and test-tube babies, gave the public the impression that science was capable of virtually anything. But for people with MS and their families, solutions were evolving much too slowly.

Nevertheless National Multiple Sclerosis Society officials tried to remain optimistic. More money was being spent on MS research than ever before, thanks to the efforts of the Society, its chapters, and the federal government. With laboratory research continuing to accelerate, Dr. H. Houston Merritt was feeling particularly optimistic in 1970 when he addressed an audience of New York business and professional leaders. Merritt, dean emeritus of Columbia University's College of Physicians and Surgeons, told the gathering, "Now there is more likelihood of making progress in MS research than at any time in the known history of the disease." Yet when the National Society commemorated its silver anniversary in 1971, it was a bittersweet occasion. It was a celebration of all that had been accomplished over the previous twenty-five years—yet progress was not fast enough for people with MS and their families who lived with the disease day after day, year after year.

The Society's efforts continued to increase public awareness of multiple sclerosis. In the ten-year period leading up to the twenty-fifth anniversary in 1971, three television networks had donated an estimated $15.7 million in free air time for educational and fundraising announcements for the Society. An equal amount of air time had been provided by local TV stations in addition to gratis public service announcements in America's magazines valued at $5 million.

During the 1970s, Society members were kept updated on the organization's activities through a number of publications—*MS Keynotes, MS Messenger,* and *MS Briefs.* These newsletters described research efforts and chapter fundraising drives, and provided profiles of people with multiple sclerosis. Yet although neither the Society nor the MS researchers could provide families with the news they wanted—that a cure was at hand—there were new reasons for genuine hope. Dr. Peter Siemens of Canada, a Society grantee, spoke at the silver anniversary conference in Los Angeles, describing his recently completed study of the natural history of multiple sclerosis. His research showed that the progression of the disease was not always as rapid or as severe as doctors had once believed. The long-term study involved seventy-four people diagnosed between 1905 and 1969, and analyzed their level of physical and social functioning; it found that 58 percent were fully active in their vocations thirty to forty years after their diagnosis.

At that anniversary conference, no one lost sight of the unfulfilled goal of the Society, and why the personal commitment of so many people remained so strong. Volunteers became even more motivated upon hearing the stories of people with multiple sclerosis like Carmen Betancourt, who at age twenty-

three told *MS Keynotes* about a dance to benefit MS research
that she had helped organize in St. Paul, Minnesota, in 1970.
The disease had already claimed the sight in her left eye, and
the vision in her right eye was weakening. But she was determined to study at a school for the blind and volunteer at the
local MS chapter because "people must know that it can happen to them." Then there were individuals like Adeline Shep-
pard, who had lived with MS for fourteen years and whose
credo was "to live as normally as possible without succumbing
to the despair that engulfs so many afflicted with a disabling
disease." She spent many hours each week tending to her gar-
den and enjoying her grandchildren, one of whom had encouraged her to "reach for the stars" with the reassuring words,
"Take a step toward me, hold my hands; I promise you, I won't
let you fall."

At that Los Angeles conference in 1971, Dr. Carl L. Ran-
dolph, chairman of the Southern California chapter, was thinking of people like Carmen and Adeline when he told the
delegates, "Let's get busy and work ourselves out of business."
His challenge was greeted with a standing ovation.

The National Society's silver anniversary was also high-
lighted by a ceremony at the White House. Sylvia Lawry,
William Breed, Jr., and Charles Meares traveled to Washington
and presented a silver tray to President Richard Nixon. The national board had given Meares the responsibility of choosing a
gift for the president. Meares chanced upon the text of a
speech given by Paul Revere, in which he described the importance of volunteerism in America. "I called the director of
Colonial Williamsburg and asked if he could make a silver tray
for us, hand wrought on Revere's own anvil," said Meares. "He
said they'd be glad to do it. On one side of the tray I had them
engrave a commemoration of the twenty-fifth anniversary of

the Society. On the reverse side they engraved Paul Revere's words."

Meares recalled the White House ceremony with some amusement, saying, "I paid for the tray myself, which was rather ironic because Nixon was one of my least favorite presidents, and I suppose I begrudged giving him a gift that I had paid for. But I kept telling myself that it was really something that I was doing for the Society, not for the president."

Meares told Nixon that the gift represented "our deep appreciation of your continuing support of volunteerism and of the Society's work." As flashbulbs exploded, he posed with the president, and many newspapers ran the photograph. As it turned out, Meares actually turned up on Nixon's infamous "enemies list," a compilation of the president's supposed political opponents that became one focus of the congressional investigation into the Nixon presidency. "I never found out how I ended up on that 'enemies list,'" said Meares, "but I guess it was because, at some point, I had given a contribution to a candidate running against Nixon."

Meares believed that at that White House event, the words spoken by the Society's entourage unwittingly became a part of another element of the Watergate scandal—the secret White House tapes. President Nixon had been running behind schedule that day, and the National Society delegation waited endlessly in the Oval Office for the president to arrive for their two o'clock appointment. "Nixon's chief of staff, Bob Haldeman, came in about every ten minutes, telling us that the president would join us shortly," Meares recalled. "But the time just dragged on and on, and finally after about an hour I turned to Bill Breed and in sort of a stage whisper said, 'I wonder if the so-and-so will ever show up!'" Two years later, Meares and the rest of the country learned that a taping system had been operating in the Oval Office beginning in 1971. It not only recorded Nixon's discussions with the Watergate principals but every other conversation in close proximity to the president's desk. "I guess my comments about Nixon became immortalized in history," said Meares.

Charles Meares was among those who believed that the governmental agency which the Society had helped create— now called the National Institute of Neurological Disorders and Stroke—wasn't being as aggressive as it might be, and needed to place MS at or near the top of its funding priorities. "The people at the Institute don't seem to take a great deal of interest in MS," he complained to colleagues. "As far as they're concerned, it's a secondary disease, because it doesn't affect as many individuals as diseases like Parkinson's."

The Society's leadership had learned that when neurologists were selecting areas in which to conduct their research, they often followed the money trail, moving in the direction of available funding. Board members believed that if they could turn multiple sclerosis into a higher-profile disease, the Institute might be more inclined to increase its funding for MS research. They wondered how they could raise the visibility of MS to get the attention of those who controlled the government's purse strings. At a subsequent board meeting, members agreed to lobby the secretary of the Department of Health, Education and Welfare (HEW) to create a commission to study MS. There had been commissions focused on other diseases, and they had heightened public and scientific interest. So why not one for MS? The board appointed Meares to spearhead the campaign to promote government interest in creating the commission. Meares led a team that began exploring tactics for stimulating support for the commission in Washington—although along the way, Meares and Sylvia Lawry clashed sharply over the best strategy to pursue.

"We were in Washington at a Society meeting, and Sylvia and I really got into it," Meares recalled. "Sylvia felt strongly that it should be a presidential commission, created by a directive from the White House. She believed that if we approached President Nixon at just the right moment, he would sign a document establishing a presidential panel. But I had been told by Congresswoman Margaret Heckler that Nixon wasn't about to do that." Sylvia had consulted Mary Lasker of the Lasker Foundation, who urged her to aim for a presidential commission because it would get much more attention and its mandate would have a greater impact.

During that long weekend in Washington, both Meares and Lawry spoke with congressional, HEW, and White House officials while also trying to reach some agreement between themselves. Meares hoped to persuade Sylvia to be more realistic, and that their best hope was to have Congress pass legislation placing the commission under the auspices of HEW. But Sylvia stood her ground, still insisting that the Society turn to the White House for support.

"We're not going to get it, Sylvia," Meares told her. "But if we direct our attention toward Congress and HEW, I've got Margaret Heckler willing to get behind this. I don't think the sponsorship—whether it's HEW or the president—matters that much."

After hours of heated argument, Sylvia finally accepted the HEW approach as the choice. Meares recalled, "She didn't approve of it, but when a decision was reached by our board, she said, 'Let's get on with it.'"

In 1972, Congress unanimously approved the establishment of the National Advisory Commission on Multiple Sclerosis. On October 25 of that year, President Nixon signed the statute forming the commission, stating that it "represents a promising step in our battle against a terrible and elusive enemy." Congress imposed the following charge on the commission: "To determine the most effective means of finding the cause and cures and treatment for multiple sclerosis," and to ascertain "the means by which the federal government can best participate in this effort."

Sylvia described the creation of the commission as "a signal achievement, one that may some day prove to have been the single most important step in the battle against MS."

Meares assumed the chairmanship of the commission, but not before miles of red tape had unwound. The White House, it seems, objected to appointing Meares to the leadership position, and had removed his name from the nominees to the commission. Heckler suspected it might be because of Meares's political affiliation.

"Are you a registered Democrat?" she asked Meares.

"No, I'm not, but what the heck does that have to do with it?"

"In this administration, everything."

"Well, I'm not a Democrat or a Republican. I'm a registered independent. Over the years I've probably given far more money to Republicans than to Democrats, but I didn't give anything to this president. In fact, I'm beginning to feel that I shouldn't give him the time of day!"

After weeks of indecision and negotiation, Meares finally was appointed chairman of the commission, and Dr. Harry Weaver was named its executive director. In all there were nine members (five scientists, four lay people) on the panel, including Dr. H. Houston Merritt. They rolled up their sleeves and got to work. Weaver, who had taken a year's leave of absence from his National Society responsibilities, called upon fifty-six of the country's leading scientists to provide assistance to the panel in evaluating the status of current research, and to shape the scientific directions that should be pursued.

The commission's work became Weaver's passion. He moved from California to Washington, D.C., and for more than a year immersed himself in a seven-day-a-week work schedule. Many months later, as the panel's work drew to a close, Weaver wrote a lengthy, detailed report—one of the most comprehensive ever to emerge from a governmental commission. When the National Advisory Commission on Multiple Sclerosis issued its final report in February 1974, the document recommended that the federal government increase its spending on MS research and basic biomedical research in the neurological sciences by $18 million above present levels during each of the following three years. The report, which was divided into twenty-seven sections, urged that research concentrate in areas such as virology, immunology, and epidemiology. Its specific recommendations included:

A concerted, collaborative effort by a task force of scientists "to work on the development and testing of therapeutic agents."

A significant push to develop an effective diagnostic test for MS.

The refinement of procedures (such as proton beam radiography and EMI scanners) that could more precisely evaluate the underlying disease process when new treatments were tested.

The creation of a comprehensive Multiple Sclerosis Treat-

ment Center to evaluate new therapies and develop approaches for reducing the sometimes disabling and painful effects (including muscle spasticity, urological difficulties,
bedsores) of MS.

The establishment of three additional government-
supported clinical research centers to facilitate the study of MS.

At a Washington press conference, Congresswoman Heckler noted that the recommended increase in MS funding would
place only a modest added burden upon taxpayers. The additional moneys amounted to less than nine cents a year for every
American. Senator Harrison Williams told the press that "the
funds recommended are very reasonable, and we will do everything we can to see that they are included in the 1975 budget."

The National Society was delighted with the report. Board
members called it "remarkable," "realistic," and "imaginative."
After Society chairman Daniel Haughton read the document,
he told HEW Secretary Caspar Weinberger, "This excellent report is most of all the brightest ray of hope to appear on the
horizon for hundreds of thousands of Americans. No one is
anticipating miracles or unjustified efforts or spending, but
anything less than a positive meaningful effort on the part of
all concerned to implement promptly the Commission's recommendations can be interpreted as a disappointment of the
cruelest dimensions."

Then the unexpected happened: the government's Neurological Disorders Institute was handed the responsibility of
implementing the report's recommendations, including ensur-
ing that money was appropriately funneled into MS research.
But Congress and the Institute dragged their feet in appropriating funds for many of the commission's recommendations.
The snail's pace of activity in Washington infuriated volunteers
and staff at the National Society. The National Society board

formally complained not only about inadequate congressional funding but also that the Institute was not spending available moneys on the specified programs.

In New York and at the chapter level, the Society launched an aggressive letter-writing campaign, urging the government to meet its MS-related commitments. "It was such a critical and very delicate period in our history," said Sylvia. "We were challenging the Neurological Institute, the very government agency that we had helped create more than two decades earlier. People whom we were dealing with at the Institute were irritated that they were being challenged in this way."

In response to the unrelenting outside pressure, the Institute finally appointed a special ad hoc advisory subcommittee to review the status of the commission's recommendations. Some members of that subcommittee claimed that inflation, especially in the medical field, had created a severe and unexpected budgetary squeeze at the Institute. Nevertheless the government gradually began making strides in carrying out the mandate of the commission, though nothing less than complete implementation could satisfy the Society. In its 1975 report, issued the following year, the National Society let some of its frustration show. It noted that the Society itself had dramatically increased its own research funding—more than doubling its allocations in 1975, compared to 1973. "The Society is meeting the challenge and, in the months to come, everything in its power will be done to ensure that the United States government does likewise."

Even today, some longtime society members point to the commission as one of the high points of the MS movement. It produced new funding for MS research and enlisted many new scientists in the search for answers to the disease. It also significantly increased public awareness of MS. Nevertheless, when

Meares looked back at what the commission had achieved, he was less than upbeat. "I guess I wasn't terribly satisfied with what we ultimately accomplished. We thought it would be much more valuable than it actually turned out to be. We believed that if we got national attention through a congressionally mandated commission, with a panel composed of eminent scientists, and spent a year laying out a plan of action, something really dramatic would come from it. But in my view it was rather disappointing because there were no real breakthroughs made on the scientific side. It really didn't go as far as we had hoped in solving the problem of MS."

Whether a presidential commission would have ensured implementation of all the recommendations is a matter of debate. Still, many of the scientists who played a part in the commission continued their commitment to MS research for many years.

25

A T FIRST GLANCE, a commitment by elite athletes to help find the cure for multiple sclerosis might seem like an unlikely scenario. In the prime of their young lives, football, baseball, and basketball stars have finely tuned bodies—quite a contrast to young people with MS, also in the prime of their lives, many of whom feel like prisoners in their own bodies. For too many individuals with MS, the struggle to take a few steps or negotiate a flight of stairs is as challenging as blasting a home run in Yankee Stadium. But what could be more touching than these sports stars—with their unique appreciation of physical coordination and balance—helping people their own age who have a serious illness that can impair bodies and shatter dreams? What could be a more humanitarian gesture than individuals with MS, many of them debilitated by their disease, being assisted by the swiftest and the strongest?

That was the thinking of Ara Parseghian, the former head football coach at the University of Notre Dame. When Parseghian played professional football for the Cleveland Browns, he was given the nickname "Hardnose" because of his fearlessness. At Notre Dame he believed that athletes had a special obligation to those whose bodies had betrayed them. Parseghian's daughter had MS, and he would eventually become a member of the National Society's Board of Directors. On the eve of the Notre Dame–Navy game in 1971, he staged a benefit for the Society. He also appeared in a sixty-second award-winning public service TV announcement for the Society, after arranging for the Ford Motor Company to donate sponsorship of the spot.

Not long thereafter, the connection between athletes and the MS movement gave the Society another big boost. The New York City chapter had been struggling in the early 1970s, with lackluster fundraising efforts that had left chapter leaders in other parts of the country asking, "If they can't raise very much money in New York, what can you expect from us?"

The national board asked Sylvia Lawry to reorganize and resuscitate the New York chapter. While she explored her options, a Society staff member and sports fan offered a suggestion: why not have a fundraising dinner for the New York chapter and invite well-known athletes as the honored guests? "I recognized the potential value of this idea immediately," said Sylvia. "It would be a way not only of raising money but of attracting new people who might eventually join the chapter board."

Sylvia convinced the national board to appropriate seed money to launch the event. It was called the MS Dinner of Champions, at which the leaders of the business community honored the outstanding athletes of the year. In 1972 the first banquet was held in New York City. Martin Davis, then the executive vice president of Gulf & Western Industries, agreed to co-chair the event; until his death in 1999, Davis continued as chairman of the New York City dinners, which were held annually. At the first banquet, Ara Parseghian received the initial MS Silver Hope Chest Award.

Though it had begun on a small scale, the Dinner of Champions strengthened the bridge between the MS community and the sports world. In the second year, Mary Wells Lawrence, head of the Wells Rich Greene advertising agency and a National Society board member, offered the services of her creative team to develop a nationwide campaign called "Athletes vs. MS." It was only one of many efforts in which the ad agency volunteered its talents.

"At the time, it was really a unique concept to incorporate athletes into the fundraising process," said national board member and treasurer John McGillicuddy. "Now it is commonplace, but I believe this was the first time that stars from the entire sports world crossed over to raise money for a good cause."

A Hall of Fame lineup of sports heroes volunteered to help. Billie Jean King, Muhammad Ali, Arnold Palmer, Tom Seaver, Henry Aaron, Lee Trevino, Jerry West, Frank Gifford, and Ara Parseghian led the parade of superstars who appeared in TV public service announcements for the Society. Gifford served as master of ceremonies of the Dinner of Champions for many years.

In 1974, Parseghian became national campaign chairman for the National Society. As the Dinner of Champions evolved into an annual affair, it rapidly became one of the most anticipated social events in New York, co-sponsored by the National Society and the city's chapter. By its third year it attracted eleven hundred guests and grossed $135,000, setting a record for a single Society-held function. The popularity of the dinner outgrew the grand ballroom of the Waldorf-Astoria Hotel, and the Society had to find larger venues, like the New York Hilton and the New York Marriott Marquis. Such superstars as Joe DiMaggio, Hank Aaron, Johnny Unitas, Rod Laver, Sugar Ray Leonard, and Peggy Fleming were honored with the MS Silver Hope Chest Award.

One businessman insisted that Sylvia personally ensure that he had tickets to the event each year, and explained the popularity of the banquet this way: "Business leaders are really just boys at heart. They love to rub shoulders with the superstars of the sports world, and get a baseball autographed by Joe DiMaggio to bring back to their sons or grandsons." At the same time Sylvia found that many of the honored athletes, conscious that their sports careers would not last forever, were eager to network with business people who might someday open doors for them in a second career.

With Martin Davis serving as national chairman, the Dinner of Champions spread to other cities. In 1974 the event raised $32,000 for the Central Pennsylvania chapter and $18,500 for the Triangle North Carolina chapter. The "Champions of Yesterday and Today" gala in Los Angeles collected $50,000.

Players from the Dallas Cowboys staged a fundraising rodeo in their city, and members of the Pittsburgh Steelers participated in the most remarkable event of all: a fashion show. Through 1978 the Dinner of Champions in cities nationwide had grossed $677,500. But that was only the beginning. In 1998 the Dinner of Champions raised more than $1.2 million for the New York City chapter alone, and the following year the dinner in Los Angeles raised a startling $3.1 million!

Sylvia felt rightfully proud of the success of these sports banquets. But the events also posed an unusual, personal challenge for her. "One year, everyone was dancing to rock and roll music at the dinner, and I was flabbergasted that I couldn't join in," she said. "So I immediately went to the Arthur Murray Dance Studio with the sole purpose of learning to dance rock and roll." Some years earlier she had won an Arthur Murray contest while dancing to the "Beer Barrel Polka," but her work for MS had kept her behind the times. So at a subsequent year's dinner, after those brush-up lessons, she spent much of the evening on the dance floor, joining the celebration to the refrains of the Beatles and the Rolling Stones.

Dances were used in other settings to raise money for the National MS Society over the years. Mary Goodyear, a prime example of the powerful volunteer, took on the project of organizing college-age men and women throughout the country. Her belief was that it made sense to start young in cultivating volunteers for multiple sclerosis—and to make these young adults aware that they could be potential victims of this disease. The "Youth Against MS" program sponsored dances and other fundraisers, and proved to be an extremely successful way to involve young people in the movement. At the same time Mary's volunteer spirit spread to her son, Charles Goodyear, an Exxon executive. Before long Sylvia had recruited Charles as a volunteer and then as a member of the executive committee of the International Federation. He also served on the Board of Directors of the National MS Society.

26

No one wanted a cure for MS more than Miriam Pepper. She grew up watching her mother's MS symptoms progressively worsen, forcing Miriam to struggle with her own feelings about her mother's increasing disability. When Miriam was in junior high school, her mom walked with the aid of a cane and with one leg dragging slightly. "Often I'd avoid being seen with my mother when she used [the cane]," Miriam wrote, "and other times the stares in public brought us closer together and made us stronger.

"High school years brought us still closer. . . . I had more responsibilities at home—all small concessions—but I fought all the way. I thought I was keeping her in line, not letting her get 'lazy' when actually she was experiencing physical weakness. We fought each other hard but reached an equilibrium. She said I kept her young and fighting."

In an article in the *St. Louis Post-Dispatch* in 1975, published shortly after Miriam had graduated from the University of California, she reflected, "Our family was optimistic and realistically oriented. Crying to [my mother] wouldn't help. So every so often, I cry alone, cry for her spirit and strength, and cry to condemn multiple sclerosis, that abominable disease."

Many other families ached for a solution to MS. They knew that every dollar raised meant that a researcher in America or overseas could pursue another scientific clue that might some-day lead to a treatment for MS. Thanks to the Society, hundreds of men and women of science were kept actively working on this formidable challenge.

In the mid-1970s, scientists studying an animal model of MS conducted early research with a mix of protein fragments—a substance called copolymer-1—taking the first steps that many years later would evolve into the MS drug Copaxone. As the decade progressed, the first computed tomography (CT) scans were performed on people with MS, providing detailed and multiple images of the human brain.

Myelin, the substance that wraps itself around nerve fibers and facilitates the transmission of nerve impulses, continued to be the focus of considerable research. Scientists thought that a complete understanding of how myelin-forming cells function might help them devise ways to prevent demyelination, or perhaps reverse the process once it had started. In the 1970s, researchers like biochemist Joseph Poduslo investigated glyco-proteins on the myelin membrane surfaces, examining whether the membranes might be susceptible to either im-munological damage or viral infection. These glycoproteins were thought to be important because they act as receptors for viruses and hormones.

Meanwhile the media were giving attention to unproven MS therapies such as snake venom and hyperbaric oxygen. A physician in Florida had been in the vanguard of administering snake venom to people with amyotrophic lateral sclerosis (ALS, or Lou Gehrig's disease), and he had begun administering the same therapy to people with MS in growing numbers. Dr. James Q. Simmons, Jr., director of medical programs for the Society, cautioned, "Aside from unsupported patient anecdotes and the doctor's own reports, there is no evidence that snake venom treatment has had any effect in either ALS or MS." Hyperbaric oxygen therapy, in which patients were exposed to pure oxygen at increased pressure, was based on one of the oldest theories of multiple sclerosis—that it is caused by a limited oxygen supply to the nervous system. But large-scale, carefully controlled studies eventually showed oxygen's ineffectiveness for treating MS.

Unlike the quick fixes promised by many promoters of unsubstantiated therapies, legitimate research can be slow, painstaking, and frustrating for those seeking a dramatic rescue from this miserable disease. But when Dr. Jonas Salk announced his decision to join the war on multiple sclerosis, there was a sense of revitalized hope among thousands of MS families. With his development of the polio vaccine, Salk had become a world-renowned celebrity, but first and foremost he saw himself as a scientist. He had already announced, "The time has arrived to find the answer to MS"—so perhaps it wasn't surprising that Dr. Harry Weaver was able to coax him into combat. Working in his research facility at the Salk Institute for Biological Studies in La Jolla, California, Salk began his MS studies with supreme expectations, believing that his dramatic success against polio would not be the only history-making story in his life.

"Our research efforts had grown considerably, but I remember how excited we were when Jonas Salk committed himself to take on MS," said John McGillicuddy, who became president of the National Society in the late 1970s. "We had been able to attract some of the better scientists, but his presence really instilled great optimism in all of us."

Dr. Salk, an immunologist by training, began studying the autoimmune process in MS. In laboratory studies, he injected a substance called myelin basic protein into animals with an MS-like illness (EAE, or experimental allergic encephalomyelitis) to see if the protein could boost immunity and control the disease. As these animal studies began, Salk showed caution in his public statements, saying, "We cannot forecast the outcome of animal experiments, nor what conclusions will be reached in respect to tests in humans."

Human studies began in early 1978. Salk injected the same myelin basic protein, produced by the Eli Lilly Research Laboratories, into people with MS. In approving the study, the U.S. Food and Drug Administration warned, "It is premature at this stage to raise false hopes," adding that this would be only "the first stage of a long testing process." As the treatments began, Salk and his co-researchers carefully monitored the condition of the volunteer subjects. Initial reports were not encouraging: there was no early evidence of improvement in people with MS. Then the unexpected happened: one of the patients died during the course of the treatment. Salk believed that the death was unrelated to the therapy and that other factors were at work. Even so, the study was abruptly ended.

Shortly thereafter Salk's life took a different turn. His enthusiasm for further MS research waned, and in the 1980s his interests shifted to AIDS. At the National Society an enormous bubble of hope had burst. Perhaps no one would have been more disappointed than Dr. Harry Weaver. But in 1977, just months before Salk's human studies began, Weaver became terminally ill with lung cancer. In the final weeks of his life, as his physical condition deteriorated and he lay in an oxygen tent, he called Sylvia Lawry almost daily from his home in California, urging her to recruit his successor immediately and even naming a few candidates. Although Sylvia was suffering from the flu and laryngitis at the time, he asked her, "What are you waiting for, Sylvia? I don't want my programs to go down the drain."

Weaver died of cancer at the age of sixty-eight. In the final weeks of his life, his belief in Salk's approach never wavered. National board chairman L. Palmer Brown observed, "In his lifetime, Dr. Weaver contributed so much to all humanity that the world, though now without him, is a far, far better place than it was before he entered it."

27

ALTHOUGH Dr. Jonas Salk's research had not found the solution to multiple sclerosis, the National Society was determined to capitalize on the scientific interest in MS that Salk
had created. The organization was able to provide researchers
with increasing funds, thanks to growing contributions, some
as small as dimes and quarters, others on an almost unimagin-
able scale. Ray Kroc, the founder of McDonald's Corporation,
while being honored at a Society banquet in Chicago, was so
moved by the event that on the spot he decided to donate $1
million to the National Society and its Chicago chapter—the
largest single gift that had ever been received. Although Kroc
was known for his generosity and had spoken publicly of his
own sister's battle with MS, the size of the contribution left
many Society staff members almost speechless. Kroc's brother
Robert, who was president of the Kroc Foundation and became
a board member of the National MS Society, explained the gift
simply and touchingly at an awards dinner in Chicago: "We can
only tell of the feeling in our hearts, that we have done good.

In this day of corporations, it is important that a corporation has a heart."

As critical as Kroc's contribution was to advancing the cause, there was something even more compelling in the money collected by many thousands of children in all parts of the nation who participated in one of the Society's most successful fundraising efforts: the MS READaTHON®. Although promoted nationwide by the National Society, it was a program run successfully by the chapters—eventually, 111 of them. It encouraged children to read—and the more they read, the more they earned for the fight against MS. In communities across America, parents, relatives, friends, and neighbors pledged nominal amounts of money—a nickel, a quarter, a dollar or more—for each book read, and when multiplied by the many youngsters who took books off shelves and enriched their lives through reading, the amounts raised by the program were phenomenal.

The READaTHON®, according to the Society's campaign literature, challenged America's children to "read for the need of others." And they certainly did. The program had been tried initially by the Northeastern Ohio Chapter in 1974, when a local board member and former teacher was looking for a way to involve children in helping the Society while benefiting themselves in the process. She brought the idea of a reading program to the Cuyahoga County Public Library Association, which endorsed it wholeheartedly. Within months the MS READaTHON® had spread throughout the country. Mrs. Lester Crown, a National Society board member from Chicago, chaired the MS READaTHON® Committee; Oscar Dystel, president of Bantam Books and another national board member, became the committee's vice chair. Dystel arranged for the back page of every Bantam book to include an application to participate in the READaTHON®.

Not surprisingly, educators loved the program, recognizing its value in motivating children to read. Instead of turning on the television set, youngsters picked up books. A film called *A New Life* was made about the READaTHON®, depicting how the program had changed the life of one child who had never before enjoyed reading but had now learned the pleasures associated with books. The imaginative program was praised not only by educators but by parents, children, librarians, and publishers.

By 1975 every Society chapter was participating in the READaTHON®. One million children had registered to participate as "Mystery Sleuths" in the program—a number that grew to 4 million in 1976. By the end of 1977, 11 million books had been read, and more than $11 million had been raised for the Society—a figure that grew to over $20 million by 1978. President Carter's daughter, Amy, was among those who participated. The program also was adopted by many MS societies abroad. Tens of thousands of children in every corner of the world developed a love of reading that could last a lifetime.

Ironically, the flood of READaTHON® money into the chapters created an unexpected dilemma. In the wake of this success, chapters suddenly had resources far beyond their projections. They began expanding, and not always judiciously. Some overextended themselves—ambitiously increasing their staffs and the services they offered, including those associated with chapter-supported MS clinics, as well as transportation and other programs. As a result, they were not always able to meet their commitments to send a share of the funds raised to the national headquarters, where at least half of it would be spent on research. Both the chapters and the National Society entered a period of adjustment and negotiation until the problem was resolved. Still, the READaTHON® was one of the Society's most rewarding programs, both for the children who read the books and for the Society volunteers who made it work. When Oscar Dystel, whose son has MS, was asked by the *MS Messenger* in 1978 how he struck the balance between the need to accept the reality of MS and the determination to work tirelessly on programs like the READaTHON®, he responded, "It isn't easy. Courage is what's needed. Renewing yourself each day so that you can prevail over the frustrations and depressions that you can't help but feel from time to time. I know that this disease is going to get licked. There's no doubt in my mind. So we must have the courage to cope with the frustrations, and the belief that the day will come."

The READaTHON® made a significant contribution toward publicizing MS. More than nine million children had enrolled in the program by 1980, making millions of Americans more aware of multiple sclerosis. "We were always looking for ways to raise the consciousness of the public about MS," said John McGillicuddy. "It was still a mystery disease to much of the public. But the READaTHON® helped change that. Now, if you mention multiple sclerosis to people, they nod. And when these young readers became adults, those coming into the medical professions were aware of this disease, the impact it was having, and the need to find a cure."

Eventually the READaTHON® was copied by other organizations, and in the competitive fundraising marketplace the National Society's program lost some of its clout. Nevertheless, it remained a remarkable success.

28

IN THE 1970s, the health of Sylvia's brother continued to deteriorate. At one point he was admitted to a community hospital with pneumonia. He had nearly recovered when his internist, just before going on vacation, recommended that Bernard be transferred to Albert Einstein Hospital to be under the care of his neurologist, Dr. Labe C. Scheinberg, who was also a member of the National Society's Medical Advisory Board. While Bernard was being transported by ambulance to Einstein Hospital, the driver became lost.

Sylvia, following behind in her car, became more and more anxious as the ambulance driver continued aimlessly down the highway. When Bernard finally arrived at the hospital, he was in a considerably weakened condition. Shortly thereafter he suffered a heart attack and died. It was a crushing blow for Sylvia and for everyone at the Society's headquarters. Bernard had lived with MS for thirty-seven years after he experienced his first symptoms. Yet on his death certificate there was no mention of multiple sclerosis. Such an omission is a common occurrence that makes death certificates unreliable sources of statistical information on MS. The death certificate was later modified by Dr. Scheinberg.

As she mourned Bernard's passing, Sylvia could have backed away from her commitment to the National Society. A few years before Bernard's death, she had also lost her husband Stanley, from her second marriage, in an automobile accident. She was a widow, raising two children on her own. "People assumed I'd lose interest in MS," she said. "In some families this does happen. But I have this obsession to find out the causes of this disease. Why did Bernard come down with it, and not me? And of course, more than anything, I want to see a cure."

After Bernard's death, thousands of cards and letters of condolence poured into the national headquarters, along with contributions in his memory. For years Sylvia could not talk about Bernard without breaking into tears. Although her brother could no longer be helped, there were hundreds of thousands of people with MS to whom Sylvia felt a commitment. Without hesitation, she continued to fight the good fight.

"Bernard loved life in whatever form he was able to live it," Sylvia said. "He had a personal goal: he wanted to be the longest survivor with multiple sclerosis. He was going to set a record. Bernard had become reconciled to the disease, believing it was his life's mission to generate hope for others with MS. His doctor felt that Bernard would have lived longer were it not for that unfortunate trip to the hospital that preceded his death.

"In an effort to boost the morale of newly diagnosed people with MS, I tell them that he survived for thirty-seven years with the disease. That's a long time—and they are reassured. And hopefully we'll finally find a cure that will help everyone who still lives with this terrible disease."

29

IN NOVEMBER 1979, Iranian militants seized fifty-three American hostages in Teheran. One of them was Richard Queen, a junior consular officer in the U.S. embassy. By the time Queen's long, painful ordeal was over, he had been diagnosed with multiple sclerosis and had become perhaps the best-known American with the disease.

For the first few weeks of his captivity, Queen felt healthy. But then he began having physical problems. He experienced slight but lingering numbness in his left arm and hand. He compared the sensations to what one might feel after plunging his hand into the snow for several minutes. When an Iranian doctor finally examined him, he told Queen, "It's nothing, it's nothing. I had the same thing once myself." Queen tried not to worry, although the symptoms persisted.

Later Queen developed itchiness on the left side of his body. The Iranian doctor gave him a supply of vitamins to "cure" his problem. But his symptoms only grew worse over the months. He became weak and dizzy. His vision blurred. He vomited frequently. After 250 days in captivity, with Iranian doctors finally acknowledging their own frustration, the militants released Queen and he was flown to Germany. At an American military base there, doctors finally diagnosed his illness as MS.

After Queen returned to the United States, he began talking freely about multiple sclerosis in media interviews. Some newspapers began referring to MS as "Richard Queen's disease." He appeared in public service announcements for the National Multiple Sclerosis Society, which also named a research fund after him. The Society's Board of Directors dedicated its 1980 Annual Report to Queen.

For every person like Richard Queen who lives with multiple sclerosis in the media spotlight, hundreds of thousands of others live quietly with the illness. In some cases even their co-workers don't know that they have MS. For others, however, the disease has overrun their bodies with such ferocity that it forces them to make major adjustments in day-to-day living that everyone around them notices. Many of them have relied on the National Multiple Sclerosis Society to champion their cause and help them live life to the fullest.

Richard Queen wasn't alone in giving multiple sclerosis greater public visibility during the early 1980s. Sylvia Lawry convinced national board member Oscar Dystel to approach Frank Sinatra, a family friend of the Dystels, and ask him to become the Society's national campaign chairman. Sinatra said, "Okay, Oscar, for you, I'll do it." Sinatra's enormous popularity helped the Society raise more than $29 million in 1981; a portion of those funds came from his benefit concert at New York's Carnegie Hall which drew a crowd of 2,800 and netted $178,000. The next year the Society raised even more—$34 million. At his own expense, Sinatra filmed TV messages in support of the Society, putting his creative input into announcements that highlighted the slogan, "FS for MS." He was also featured on 10,000 subway posters for the organization.

When Sinatra received the National Hope Chest Award as the Outstanding Volunteer of the Year for 1981 at a banquet in Houston, he told the large audience that he had not been fully aware of the potentially devastating nature of MS. "But when I was exposed to it, I realized what it takes to go on with this kind of ailment, this terrible disease," he said. "I've been involved with lots of causes. Yet there's so much passion with regard to MS in the people I've met. They've touched me dearly and deeply." Sinatra had been the best man at the wedding of Oscar Dystel's son, John. Sinatra said, "John is afflicted with MS, and he is so courageous. I thought to myself, I wonder if I would have enough guts to take a chance on marriage at such a time in my life, being incapacitated as he was. It was very moving."

Whenever Sinatra appeared at a National MS Society event, he paid his own expenses to get there. And if he was faced with a scheduling conflict, he made sure that someone was there to represent him—often his wife, Barbara. When Sinatra was unable to attend a Society event at the White House, he chartered a plane and flew Barbara and Sylvia Lawry from New York to Washington. As the two women ate lunch while airborne, Sylvia was cutting a small plum tomato on her plate when the tomato burst open, squirting its juice all over Barbara's dress.

Sylvia was abashed. "There we were, on our way to the White House, and I had splattered tomato juice all over her," she said. "I was so embarrassed." Barbara Sinatra was unfazed. She proceeded to clean the dress as best she could. They arrived at the White House with Barbara's clothes just a little worse for wear, and they met with President Reagan, tomato stains and all. "She kept telling me, 'Don't worry about it,'"

Sylvia recalled. "I felt much worse than she did." Their friend-ship remained untainted by the tomato incident.

Frank Sinatra served as national campaign chairman for three years.

30

SYLVIA LAWRY and the National MS Society have always been inseparable. From its humble origins in the one-room office at the Academy of Medicine building, to the more expansive headquarters on Forty-second Street that became the Society's offices as the 1980s began, Sylvia Lawry nurtured the Society's growth from her executive director's chair.

But there were worrisome signs in the early 1980s. In the 1981 Annual Report, National Society Chairman Norman Cohn and President Ralph Weller called that year a "trial by fire" period for all nonprofit organizations. "A tight economy and a marked decrease in federal funds have put their survival to a crucial test," they wrote. "The National Multiple Sclerosis Society has responded to this challenge with vigor, creativity and growth—a tribute to the enthusiasm and determination at both national and chapter levels of our dedicated volunteers and staffs."

By 1982 the national board began considering bringing in new management to chart the organization's future path toward new growth. Some board members believed that the Society could raise more money. Proceeds from the READ-aTHON® had begun to plateau, and some board members questioned whether the launching of a door-to-door solicitation campaign was the most effective use of manpower.

At the same time Sylvia began to experience health problems of her own. She had frequent bouts of flu and allergies, which appeared to be related to the stress associated with overseeing both the national and international MS movements. She became concerned about her own well-being, and so did her fellow board members. To keep up with the times and ensure that the Society moved forward, the board ultimately made one of its toughest decisions ever: it voted to create a search committee, headed by Clifford Goldsmith, then the president of Philip Morris USA, to find and hire a president and CEO to assume leadership of the Society.

With the help of an executive search firm, the board identified the leading candidate, retired Vice Admiral Thor Hanson. Less than a year earlier, Hanson had retired from the navy after a thirty-one-year career that had begun when he graduated from the U.S. Naval Academy in 1950 with a degree in engineering. He went on to win a Rhodes scholarship to Oxford University in England, where he studied philosophy, politics, and economics. As a naval officer he commanded eight cruisers and fifty destroyers, and served as military assistant to Secretary of Defense Harold Brown, aide to Secretary of the Navy John Chafee, and a systems analyst in the office of the defense secretary.

In 1982, Hanson was a commentator for CNN in Washington, D.C. With three of his five children still in high school, he was unsure about moving his family to New York. But after being formally offered the job, he accepted the challenge. On November 1, 1982, when Hanson met with the National MS

Society staff for the first time as the Society's new president and CEO, he stepped into the conference room and told the gathering, "I retired as vice admiral because I wanted time to have a substantive second career to which I could bring a sense of dedication, but also one in which I—and you—could have some fun." At six feet four inches, with an engaging smile and an easy laugh, Hanson quickly won the confidence of the group. He readily admitted that when first approached about the job he hadn't known much about multiple sclerosis, nor had the disease struck anyone in his family. But as he had proven in the navy, Hanson was a quick learner and had a strong sense of purpose. When its leadership was passed from Sylvia Lawry to Hanson, the National Society issued a news release that said simply: "Thor Hanson was elected President and Chief Executive Officer of the National Multiple Sclerosis Society. He succeeds Sylvia Lawry, who becomes Founder-Director. She will devote herself, on the Society's behalf, to the International Federation of Multiple Sclerosis Societies and the National Committee on Neurological and Communicative Disorders."

In the National Society's 1982 Annual Report, dedicated to Sylvia Lawry, she remarked: "To everything there is a season. In Admiral Hanson we have found a person who can ensure continuity and performance. This leaves me free, 'unfettered,' as Board member Palmer Brown puts it, to impact on other spheres which I think can move us more swiftly toward our goals. The time is right for this next step, just as the time proved right (in 1945) to put that ad in the *Times*."

Nevertheless Sylvia relinquished her leadership of the National Society with some trepidation. Like her sons Frank and Steven, the Society was one of her children. It was an organization she had nurtured from its birth. Though she felt excitement taking on the challenge of managing the international interests of the National MS Society, while continuing to serve on the Society's board and working as a volunteer for the International Federation, she knew that the Society had ongoing problems to solve, and initially she did not know what to expect under the new regime.

"I had been managing a tremendous load," Sylvia said. "I was responsible for the National Society and building the International Federation and the national Societies abroad in my 'spare time.' I had developed respiratory and allergy problems, and my health status was very troubling." Her doctor, in fact, warned Sylvia that she was "digging an early grave" and should ease up for her own good.

Sylvia knew that she still had plenty of ideas to contribute. Now the International Federation became the primary beneficiary of her energy. "I had less overall responsibility and less stress, and as a result my health improved," she said. "It also gave me more time to help develop the international movement."

In the 1982 Annual Report, the dedication page flowed with kind words for Sylvia, conveying the board's "deep love and profound admiration for history already made in the world health movement. In seeking a single candlepower of light for one beloved person, she has illuminated the lives of hundreds of thousands of MS persons throughout the world. We also recognize she is not at the end of her journey . . . merely at the beginning of another."

If Sylvia felt any concerns about how her colleagues would react to her shift of responsibilities, those concerns were quieted as she opened her mail in the ensuing weeks. Her desk overflowed with letters of praise, many from the nation's leading neurologists.

"If I could select a single word to epitomize what you have done, it would be to point out that you truly have brought *hope* to individuals with MS, and to their families and friends. The organization which you evolved stands as a model of what a voluntary health organization should be, and I believe it is unique among such organizations in the arena of the clinical neurosciences." —Dr. Donald H. Silberberg, Chair and Professor of Neurology, University of Pennsylvania.

"No other layman has done more for the cause of neurological science and the solution to crippling and progressive disorders. I have had tremendous respect for your energy, intelligence, and determination in the work that you carried out for the Society, and have used you as a model of what the intelligent lay person can accomplish when that person teams up with science in the cause of humanity." —Dr. Fred Plum, Chair and Professor of Neurology, Cornell University Medical College.

"Your efforts have been unique and will be long remembered by everybody associated with the MS cause. As I am sure you are aware, there are legions of patients and MS investigators who will be forever indebted to you." —Dr. Kenneth P. Johnson, Chair and Professor of Neurology, University of Maryland School of Medicine.

"If ever a great organization belonged to one person, this one belonged to you. In my entire medical career, I have not encountered anyone with your singleness of purpose and dedication to this kind of altruistic, humanitarian and scientific goal. I never ceased marveling at your optimistic conviction that the goal would ultimately be won, nor to be amazed at the unflagging tenacity of will with which you spurred on the fighters in the greater battle. . . . The National Multiple Sclerosis Society was, is, and as long as you live, always will be, 'your baby.'"

—Dr. George A. Schumacher, Emeritus Professor of Neurology, University of Vermont College of Medicine.

Sylvia also enjoyed more formal recognition. She visited the White House to accept the President's Volunteer Action Award, which recognized her service to the community. She also received the Distinguished Service Award from the National Health Council.

Admiral Hanson often recognized the enormous challenge he faced in following in Sylvia's footsteps. "One never replaces such a unique person," he said. "One only builds on the solid and significant foundations she has had the wisdom and ability to provide. This is my aim."

31

W HEN I took office," Thor Hanson said, "the Society had not been able to fund some of the research it had hoped to support. It was a fact that we were not keeping pace with the other outstanding health organizations; it was a fact that we needed to take a close look at ourselves."

The research budget for the upcoming year, which had been projected at $6 million, actually topped out at $5.7 million, meaning that several new grants could not be approved for funding. Hanson immediately instituted a reorganization effort that would make more funds available for research. His restructuring included some difficult cuts in staff at the national office. "Reorganization can be painful," he said, "but when we can announce that we have been able to fund additional research, the effort will have been worth it."

There were changes in the chapters as well. "In any big organization," said Hanson, "you always have turf problems, where individuals in the chapters think, 'The people at the national headquarters don't know what's going on out here.' So we worked hard to reduce the friction between the chapters and the national." Clifford Goldsmith formed a Chairman's Advisory Council of chapter chairpersons, which began meeting annually with members of the national staff to improve communication and cooperation. In 1983, Hanson set another goal: to reduce the number of chapters from 135 to 90 by the end of the decade—a goal that he ultimately reached. Inefficient chapters, he said, needed to be combined with nearby chapters that were functioning at a higher level. This consolidation, he believed, would streamline local operations, reduce overlap, and resolve some of the chapter problems that existed. "This process is never easy, because local boards don't like to be merged," said Hanson. "But we just have to do it to get rid of the inefficiency where we see it. At the same time, we also want to form branches of some of the larger existing chapters."

The national headquarters also gave greater recognition to the importance of programs on the local level, from support groups to local referrals to employment workshops. Research, of course, remained a chief priority too, with Hanson calling the work of the scientific community "the key to the solution of medical problems—specifically, the cause and cure of multiple sclerosis." But the national office also made every effort to ensure that those who provided day-to-day services knew how much they were appreciated. While there were only about twenty chapters with service directors in 1983, often because of financial constraints, the national board began providing subsidies so that local directors could help other chapters strengthen their programs. At the same time, improvements in wheelchairs, lifts, accessible vans, and electric door openers— plus the increasing availability of computers—made life better for individuals with MS.

In the mid-1980s, Donald Tykeson joined the Society's Board of Directors, bringing his unique perspective of a person

with MS to the governing body. Since Henry J. Kaiser, Jr.'s service on the board in the late 1940s, people with the disease had
frequently participated in the organization's leadership ranks,
but few came to the organization like Tykeson.

When he was diagnosed in his twenties, Tykeson was told
by his physician, "You'll probably wind up in a wheelchair
someday, but it's hard to say how soon." For many years Tykeson had a practice of starting each calendar year by writing
down his top ten objectives for the coming twelve months. For
years his list included the goal of becoming involved with the
National MS Society—but it was always something he put off
until an unusual sailing trip along the Columbia River in the
Pacific Northwest, which he shared with people active in the
Society.

"The boat unexpectedly got stuck in a sandbar a mile from
shore," said Tykeson. "For four hours I was a captive audience."
The lobbying was good-natured but intense, and by the time
the boat was freed, Tykeson had agreed to become the MS activist that he had always felt he should be.

Hanson and the entire board challenged the National Society to reach out to more people with multiple sclerosis and
their families. "In 1983 we were reaching perhaps 25 percent
of those who had MS," he said. "I hoped that 75 percent would
be interfacing with the Society."

To achieve that goal, the Society tried increasing its visibility through outreach efforts. The organization obtained a
grant to establish an Information Resource Center (IRC),
which became a comprehensive clearinghouse of information
about MS. Its diverse resources included medical journals, textbooks, scientific reports, articles in the popular press, and materials written for people with MS and their families. Early on,
the IRC entered the world of computerized databases, in which

information could be located almost instantaneously to respond to inquiries from physicians and the public about MS diagnosis, symptoms, treatments, and psychosocial issues.

The Society also created a national toll-free telephone line that began fielding dozens of calls daily from individuals asking for general and specific information about the disease and how best to live with it. Board member Oscar Dystel was the driving force behind the creation of the toll-free service. Just weeks after it was inaugurated, more than four thousand calls were received and handled within a ten-day period in response to a widely publicized *New England Journal of Medicine* article on MS drug development. Over the years the toll-free line and the Information Resource Center became definitive sources of MS information—so much so that, according to Hanson, "If you call the government's National Institute of Neurological Disorders and Stroke and ask a question about MS, they'll refer you to the National Multiple Sclerosis Society."

The year 1983 also saw the debut of *Inside MS*, a new quarterly magazine for members of the Society. Although it wasn't the organization's first publication, its twenty-four pages were published in a large format—with larger type, larger photos and easier handling for people with MS, many of whom had vision problems. It described the lives of "doers" in the movement, activities of the national office and the chapters, research programs, progress in medical treatments, government legislation, and services for persons with MS.

Changes also came about in the Society's research effort. Dr. Byron Waksman emerged as the successor to Henry Weaver to direct the organization's research programs. Waksman was an immunologist, microbiologist, and bench scientist, and an early recipient of a National MS Society grant. He had conducted research at both Harvard and Yale and was excited by a scientific challenge as complex as multiple sclerosis. Research was in his blood: he had grown up with a father who was a Nobel laureate. Dr. Selman Abraham Waksman had discovered streptomycin, the first antibiotic effective in the battle against tuberculosis. His son Byron cultivated his own scientific curiosity while washing beakers and observing the workings of his father's lab at Rutgers University. The elder Waksman, a renowned scientist, routinely worked late into the night, wearing a white smock that had holes at both elbows. When asked about the smock, the elder Waksman said, "It's a disgrace to my secretary, my wife, and the university. But it serves the purpose."

Dr. Byron Waksman was more likely to wear sleeveless sweaters. He smiled frequently, but there was intensity behind the grin that served him and the Society well as he led the next phase of the war on MS. Much of Waksman's energy was directed toward the immunological aspects of MS and the possibility that a viral infection, perhaps in the early years of life, might be the cause of the disease. A virus, Waksman knew, might remain hidden in cells of the nervous system for the rest of an individual's life, and like the herpes virus that causes cold sores or the chickenpox virus that erupts as shingles, it might reexpress itself years later. He promised to investigate "the possibility that immune reactions to a virus, intended primarily for defense, may themselves damage tissue and produce disease. In this case, the nervous system tissues would represent innocent bystanders caught in the battle and destroyed by forces attempting to protect them." Some investigators believed that Waksman was putting too much emphasis on immunology in MS research, and argued that more research dollars should be awarded in other areas.

In the 1980s, funds were supporting 113 projects by American men and women of science who were working to solve the mysteries of MS. When Waksman formally took on his new position in 1979, he said, "The scientists working under Society grants are first rate. They are as good as you'll find. They are innovative and dedicated, and like good scientists everywhere, they are motivated by curiosity."

In cooperation with the International Federation of Multiple Sclerosis Societies, Waksman wrote the first edition of *Therapeutic Claims in Multiple Sclerosis,* an invaluable, authoritative resource for people with MS and their physicians. First published in 1982 and updated every few years since, Waksman and his successors have reviewed current MS treatments—conventional, unproven, and pure quackery—offered in the United States and abroad. They have described and evaluated drugs, chemical preparations, diets, and surgical procedures. With advice from a committee of experts, the book has explained the rationale behind each treatment, the claims and the research surrounding it, and reached a conclusion on the risks and benefits of the therapy.

On other fronts, the first magnetic resonance imaging (MRI) of the cranial plaques of MS was performed in 1981. An MRI could reveal up to ten times as many lesions in the brain as any other technique, and rapidly became a cornerstone of diagnosis. Before the end of the decade, sequential MRI scans had proven that multiple sclerosis is a constantly active disease, though symptoms may not always be present. Meanwhile the International Federation and the National Multiple Sclerosis Society sponsored a global conference that confirmed double-blind, placebo-controlled clinical trials as the gold standard for testing new treatments in MS.

To the doomsayers frustrated by the complexity of MS that consistently thwarted hopes for a breakthrough, Waksman often quoted Macfarland Burnet, a Nobel laureate who in 1949 declared, "I see no hope of a poliomyelitis vaccine being produced." A short time later Dr. Jonas Salk, building on a growing body of research, developed a lifesaving vaccine. Discussing multiple sclerosis, Waksman observed, "Our advance seems 'slow' to outsiders, but it is steady, it is continuous, and right now it is exciting." He told a National Society conference, "The MS problem is going to be solved, quite possibly within the lifetimes of the oldest people in this audience, and I hope while I'm still holding this job."

32

ONCE Thor Hanson assumed leadership of the National MS Society, Sylvia Lawry turned her full attention to the International Federation of Multiple Sclerosis Societies (IFMSS). With all of her energies now directed globally, she could even more effectively help the worldwide movement grow, serving as the Federation's secretary and a member of its nominating committee.

As word spread that Sylvia was stepping aside as executive director of the National Society, however, some international MS leaders were disturbed by the changes in the power structure at the New York headquarters. Kunio Izumi was one of them. The president of one of the largest exporting companies in Japan, he had never heard of multiple sclerosis when he first met Sylvia. But he soon became so committed to the cause that he devoted two years of his life to establishing an MS society in Japan. When he met with Sylvia at her office, and she confirmed that she was resigning, he was clearly upset. "We don't do such things in Japan," Izumi told her. "You recruited me. If you resign from the MS movement, it naturally follows that I will resign, too. You should have come to me first and discussed this with me."

Sylvia was a little startled, but she assured Izumi that she had no intention of abandoning her dedication to the movement. She would only be shifting gears and directing her attention to the International Federation now. Izumi smiled. He appeared greatly relieved. They shook hands, and he told her that his own commitment would remain as strong as ever. "My goal," he said, "is for the cure for MS to come from Japan." She responded, "More power to you."

Over the years, Sylvia was only one of the many heroes of the international movement. Rome Betts, an early secretary-general of the IFMSS, had been executive director of the American Heart Association and president of the National Health Council. "Betts knew all the ins and outs of the voluntary health agency movement, and I thought he'd be perfect for the job," said Sylvia. He was succeeded by Sidney O'Donoghue, the son of a U.S. Foreign Service officer. O'Donoghue had been raised in Europe and Latin America, and during his tenure with the International Federation he lived in Vienna and visited countries throughout the world, helping to create and strengthen new national societies in Finland, Israel, Argentina, and Chile, among others. His trip to Australia launched a $1 million research fund drive in a country where the emphasis had traditionally been on services.

Although Sylvia's attention never strayed far from her focus of stimulating research throughout the world, she also never lost sight of the beneficiaries of that research—people with MS and their families. The IFMSS established the International Group of MS Persons, then created an award honoring the International MS Person of the Year, a prize similar to one already being given to Americans by the National MS Society. "The concept of the award is that by honoring the out-standing personal achievements of people with MS, this will help dispel the defeatist feelings among many persons with the disease who feel they can no longer make plans for the future," said Sylvia. Competition among countries for the International MS Person of the Year Award became so fierce, and the back-lash against certain award winners became so heated, that the protocol for selecting the recipient had to be modified. Factors in addition to personal achievement became part of the crite-ria for choosing the award winner, including the individual's involvement with the national Society of the country in which he or she lived.

One of the best-known international personalities ever to battle MS was Jacqueline du Pre. When she experienced the first symptoms of multiple sclerosis, she thought she was losing her mind. A British-born prodigy in her early teens who had be-come one of the world's most brilliant cellists, du Pre believed that her active imagination might be sabotaging her body, and she sought help from a psychiatrist. One afternoon, as she re-hearsed for a concert with Leonard Bernstein and the New York Philharmonic Orchestra, she couldn't feel the cello strings nor properly maneuver her bow. She told Bernstein she couldn't play that night, but he wouldn't listen. Believing she was just nervous, he convinced her to perform. She walked onto the stage with weakened arms and numb fingers. She played the best she could. Not surprisingly, however, her per-formance was substandard. Immediately after the concert, Bernstein took her to a doctor. The diagnosis? Stress.

Seven long months later, Jacqueline du Pre's illness was fi-nally identified as MS. Overnight she became one of the world's most famous people with the disease. The headline on the front page of London's *Daily Mail* read "Jacqueline du Pre Will Never Play in Public Again."

In the mid-1970s, Jacqueline began chasing experimental therapies, many of them suggested in letters from well-meaning fans. She swallowed megavitamins. She tried acupuncture treatments. She traveled to the Rockefeller Institute in New York where researchers were analyzing blood samples on the theory that MS might be related to the measles virus. Meanwhile Jacqueline was forced to abandon her performing career. She became a cello teacher at her home in London, giving private lessons and master classes for students who arrived from all over the world. One of them was James Wolfensohn, an international investment banker and partner at Salomon Brothers with a great love of music, who had become a friend of Jacqueline and her husband, Daniel Barenboim. Personally devastated by the toll that multiple sclerosis had taken on his cello instructor, Wolfensohn joined with Barenboim in creating a foundation in her honor to support research in MS. At the time they weren't aware of the MS Society of Great Britain and Northern Ireland, nor of the International Federation. Later, when Jacqueline became involved with the MS Society in the UK, it was the first time she had ever met another person with the disease.

Jacqueline agreed to attach her name to a series of fundraising concerts that would benefit the Jacqueline du Pre Research Fund, and the first one was held in London. Sylvia Lawry contacted Wolfensohn and tried to persuade him that the International Federation would be an ideal vehicle for sponsoring those concerts. She described the volunteer strength of the member societies and how they could help fill the seats at the concerts and raise money for MS research.

Wolfensohn listened and liked what he heard. He recognized that the IFMSS could advance the cause, so he accepted the Federation's offer of support.

The first du Pre concert under the sponsorship of the Federation, featuring Russian emigré pianist Vladimir Ashkenazy, attracted a capacity audience to Carnegie Hall in New York. It netted nearly $100,000, 90 percent of which went directly into research, with the remaining 10 percent supporting the operations of the International Federation. Subsequent concerts featured classical musicians—including Artur Rubinstein, Itzhak Perlman, Zubin Mehta, and Pinchas Zukerman and his wife— all of whom donated their time, allowing the money raised to be channeled directly into MS research.

At one point Sylvia flew to London to meet with Jacqueline du Pre at her home. The famed cellist greeted her warmly, and they spent about two hours together. Jacqueline was in a wheel-chair, and her illness had progressed to a point where she sometimes had difficulty speaking clearly. Sylvia asked her, "Do you think that all the professional pressures and strains you were exposed to early in your life played any role in the development of MS?" Jacqueline's answer surprised her. "The pressure was never a problem for me. I loved every minute of it. I wouldn't have had it any other way." As Sylvia was about to leave, Jacqueline wistfully asked her, "Do you think I will be remembered after I'm gone?" Sylvia responded, "Of course. We will see to that." Jacqueline was extraordinarily pleased.

Later Jacqueline told a newspaper reporter, "We still can't be sure that I will never play again. Nobody knows if I'll ever regain mobility. It could be that next week I'll find myself walking down the road. I believe in realistic optimism but not wishful thinking."

Today the du Pre Fellowship provides funds for young scientists and clinicians from developing countries, enabling them to pursue research and work with some of the world's leading MS investigators. The fellowship is providing more short-term exchange visits by researchers than ever before. In 1999, Leonard Slatkin, the acclaimed conductor and music director of the National Symphony Orchestra in Washington, D.C., became chairman of the du Pre Research Fund. At the same time he agreed to become an ambassador for the MS cause, hoping to expand public awareness of the disease. When he accepted the leadership role with the du Pre Research Fund, he said, "Jackie's contribution to the world of music was phenomenal, and as she fought MS she brought worldwide attention to the plight of everyone battling the devastating effects of this disease. I am very proud and truly honored to have this opportunity to serve as chair of the Jacqueline du Pre MS Research Fund."

James Wolfensohn's friendship with Jacqueline du Pre led to something even more significant than the du Pre benefit concerts. Sylvia had been extremely impressed with his personal integrity and strong interest in multiple sclerosis. She recognized that if the International Federation could tap into the leadership skills of the Australian-born Wolfensohn, the movement would take a quantum leap toward its goal of solving the mysteries of MS. She decided to try to persuade the investment banker to fill the impending vacancy of the presidency of the federation. But the IFMSS wasn't the only organization seeking Wolfensohn's talents. Among other positions, he would become president of the World Bank, chairman of the Board of New York's Carnegie Hall, and chairman of the board of trustees of the John F. Kennedy Center for the Performing Arts in Washington, D.C. In 1995 he was awarded an honorary knighthood by Queen Elizabeth II for his contribution to the arts.

Wolfensohn seriously considered Sylvia's offer. Then, in a meeting with her and national board members Charles Meares and Joseph Monge (vice president of the International Paper Corporation) he told Sylvia, "I'll do it as long as you can assure me that I won't be a dark horse, and that there will be no opposition to my candidacy." She believed that was a promise she could confidently make, particularly after she had canvassed all the members of the Federation's nominating and executive committees. Although most did not know Wolfensohn personally, they agreed that he would be an ideal candidate. One by one, they committed their support for him. With Sylvia's reassurance, Wolfensohn agreed to have his name placed before the next meeting of the International Federation in Amsterdam and to go through the process of being elected the organization's next president.

"It's a coup to have Wolfensohn interested in the presidency," Sylvia had told her colleagues. She vowed to him that his election would not be contested—but she was unaware that another candidate was being considered for the top spot by some delegates at the conference site in Amsterdam. In fact the stage was set for an all-out war for the presidency of the International Federation—and plenty of embarrassment for Sylvia when Wolfensohn's candidacy was considered and resisted.

When Wolfensohn was confronted with cross-examination at the conference, he became furious. He called for a recess and told Sylvia, "Either you have been deceived, or you have deceived me! I'm of a mind to take the next plane home!"

Sylvia felt chagrined and humiliated. It was one of the most painful moments of her long experience in the MS move-

ment. She assured Wolfensohn that she had not misrepre-
sented the fact that all bases had been touched. She remained
convinced that he would be a great asset as president—and was
delighted when he decided to address the delegates directly
from the podium. It was a dramatic event in the history of the
International Federation. Before a hushed audience, Wolfensohn talked firmly and passionately. He spoke about Jacqueline
du Pre. He described his own determination to discover the answers to MS. He moved the audience. He motivated them. And
he won the support of the delegates. He was unanimously
elected president.

During his six-year tenure at the helm of the Federation,
Wolfensohn did not disappoint. He created unparalleled harmony among the member societies and strengthened their support for the IFMSS. When he relinquished his presidential
gavel, several people approached Sylvia and asked, "Where will
we ever find another Jim Wolfensohn?"

Fortunately, as president emeritus, Wolfensohn remained
an active member of the executive committee for many years.
His successors carried impressive credentials of their own, including George C. Boddiger, his immediate successor. Boddiger grew up on a family farm, and his father had hoped that he
would take over the operation someday. But George had his
sights set on the business world, and he eventually became
president and CEO of the Equitable Life Insurance Company
in Washington, D.C. Although he had no multiple sclerosis in
his own family, Boddiger's compassion translated into more
than three decades of commitment to conquering MS. After
several leadership positions on the chapter and national levels—including chairman of the Los Angeles chapter and a
member of the boards of the Washington chapter and the National Society—he became intrigued with the international

program and served as one of its most respected presidents. "He had never heard of MS when he first got involved," said Sylvia. "But he has so much expertise and talent that an agency such as ours benefits from, and that money can't buy. He has been an invaluable adviser to me on thousands of occasions. I still find him helpful as a sounding board, as did the presidents who succeeded him."

Boddiger's successor was William Benton, an executive with the Ford Motor Company, whose involvement with the MS movement dated to his pinch-hitting as chairman of the Dinner of Champions in New York one year when Martin Davis was unable to host the event. In his closing remarks at the dinner, Benton mentioned that Ford was sending him to London to oversee the auto manufacturer's operations in Europe. Dan Haughton, who was seated next to Sylvia at the banquet, leaned over and whispered to her, "Go after him, Sylvia, for the International Federation." And that's what she did. For years Benton enjoyed telling the story that Sylvia was waiting for him at the airport in London upon his arrival there. He agreed to become involved in the movement, and on his own initiative began raising funds for the MS Society in the United Kingdom. Before long he had assumed the presidency of the International Federation.

From the earliest days of the National MS Society, Sylvia Lawry routinely spread herself thin, taking on many more responsibilities than she could reasonably fit into a twenty-four-hour day. That didn't change once her attention shifted to the International Federation. She often lived out of a suitcase, traveling from one country to another to help launch or stimulate the expansion of the National Society there. On a visit to Mexico City in 1984, she met with Mexico's most influential neurologist, Dr. Manuel Velasco-Suarez, then director of that country's Neurological Institute. While there she also encouraged fifteen leading neurologists and neuroscientists to serve on the first Medical Advisory Board of the new Mexican MS Society. She was highly persuasive; all of them agreed to participate. National Society board member Clifford H. Goldsmith also arranged for her to confer with key business people in Mexico, many of whom joined the Board of Directors of the Mexican Society. Goldsmith invited William Tiernay, a Philip Morris executive responsible for Mexico, to assist her, and by the time Sylvia's two-month stay in Mexico had ended, the new board was composed of an array of prominent citizens. She even recruited Cantinflas, an actor (*Around the World in 80 Days*) and a national hero of Mexico, to serve on the board and to appear in TV spots appealing for funds.

The most influential volunteer in the Mexican MS Society became Adolfo Autrey. He is a member of one of the leading families of Mexico and a successful businessman in the pharmaceutical and other important industries. Yet he became president of the national MS Society there almost by default. During Sylvia's two-month visit to Mexico, no one would accept the presidency of the new Society, and she finally told the new board members, "I'm not going to leave Mexico until someone agrees to become president!" To ensure continuity, Autrey finally gave in. "I'll be president until you find someone else," he said. As the twentieth century drew to a close, he was not only still president but had joined the International Federation's Board of Directors. Even though there was no one with MS in his family, Autrey's sense of responsibility to the cause has been unwavering.

33

W HEN SYLVIA returned to the United States from a trip abroad, her pace rarely slowed. At one point, she approached officials at the Hilton Foundation and convinced them to award a two-year grant to pay for the IFMSS's publication of quarterly reports designed to keep member societies and researchers abreast of scientific studies and advances in multiple sclerosis. Dr. Byron Waksman, a driving force behind MS research in the United States, expanded his own mission to work on behalf of the International Federation to stimulate global research. He chaired the scientific programs committee of the International Federation and, as a way to encourage MS research, staged a series of scientific workshops, supported by the Federation, its member societies, and the U.S. government's National Institute of Neurological Disorders and Stroke. Scientists from around the world attended the workshops to discuss ongoing research and directions worthy of pursuing in the future. Later, satellite conferences were inaugurated, held in conjunction with the Federation's annual meeting, to disseminate research findings to scientists everywhere.

Concurrently there was real innovation in the MS service programs in many countries. In the United Kingdom, the MS Society of Great Britain and Northern Ireland established Holiday Homes throughout the UK. Each one was a fully equipped vacation and respite facility, designed to meet the unique needs of people with MS and their families. Instead of a hospital-like environment, these retreats were estates and country manors converted into recreational facilities, providing opportunities for socialization, and staffed with health-care professionals who could provide medical care for people with MS. They were financed largely through the government's nationalized health program.

A similar program was launched in Denmark, sponsored by the Danish MS Society. Ernst Klaebel, then owner of the leading Danish newspaper and a member of the International Federation's board, had forty-two houses built on beachfront property in that country, with the help of government subsidies. Each home was wheelchair accessible and had a kitchen unit and other amenities especially designed for the needs of people with MS. Wheelchair ramps led right down to the beach. The homes in Denmark allowed people with MS and their entire families to enjoy a vacation together at reasonable prices.

The MS Society in Sweden, along with the government of that country, developed a program in the Canary Islands where persons with MS were able to vacation during the chilly Swedish winters. Some of these facilities combined recreational programs with rehabilitation.

Meanwhile the MS Society in France borrowed the concept of the successful Dinner of Champions from the National MS Society in the United States and its chapters—the first time the fundraising event was held outside North America. With the encouragement of the International Federation, the banquet was staged in Bordeaux and brought together leading athletes from throughout Europe, raising the equivalent of 200,000 U.S. dollars for the French Society. Since then the dinner has been repeated in Lyon, Nantes, and Toulouse.

At about the same time, James Cantalupo, who served as president of the International Federation, helped spread interest in the MS READaTHON® program to many parts of the world. Cantalupo, who has a sister with MS, is also vice chairman of the McDonald's Corporation. He approached Coca-Cola and convinced the soft drink company to provide a major grant over a three-year period to support the Federation's READaTHON® programs.

In Belgium the MS Society raised the equivalent of $3 million through a Swim-Marathon, an event held in fifty pools throughout the country on a single weekend. "So often," said Sylvia, "I've heard that fundraising in Europe can never be expected to reach the levels of the U.S. But the Swim-Marathon in Belgium showed that the potential is there to match the levels at home. It is very exciting and encouraging to see what is being accomplished in so many countries. We are exporting our form of volunteerism, providing for lay leadership, supported by advisory medical and scientific leaders. This has been catching on."

Despite these kinds of successes, the International Federation has often had to deal with financial crises of its own. Because membership dues do not cover even the IFMSS's operating costs, funds must be raised continuously to meet the most basic expenses of the organization. One of the most unusual of those fundraisers was a reception at No. 11 Downing Street in London to commemorate International Multiple Sclerosis Year in 1993. Proceeds from the event were shared by the

IFMSS and the MS Society of Great Britain and Northern Ireland.

As the twenty-fifth anniversary of the IFMSS approached, the Federation appointed a silver jubilee committee to oversee the commemoration of that landmark event. The committee decided to use the anniversary to increase public awareness of MS, and in the process to help the International Federation's member societies boost their own fundraising efforts. In most national societies, research continued to take a back seat to services, and there were hopes by many International Federation officials that the heightened attention on MS might stimulate more government appropriations for research. Nevertheless, even today, England, Canada, Australia, the Netherlands, Denmark, and the United States are the only countries with aggressive research campaigns.

"In fact, in 1999, our own National MS Society in the U.S., and the society in the United Kingdom, were the only national societies that had a full-time research director in charge of overseeing their research efforts," said Sylvia. "In most countries they were guided by a volunteer Medical Advisory Board chairman who was often a practicing neurologist and was more geared toward delivering clinical services to people with MS. Of course, it's quite a responsibility to provide service, and that's where the priority had been placed."

As new national MS Societies were formed, the number of member societies in the International Federation continued to grow. By 2000 the number of member societies had grown to thirty-eight. The MS movement spread to Russia, Pakistan, Lebanon, Venezuela, Colombia, Lithuania, Estonia, Ukraine, Cuba, Chile, and Panama. Particularly in the Eastern European countries, however, medical care and services for people with MS are very limited. "It's hard to imagine the wonder of the

Eastern European delegates when they attend our international conferences," said Sylvia. "It boggles their minds to see what is available in other countries for people with multiple sclerosis. They're so strapped for money and resources; they don't have even the fundamentals, like wheelchairs for people who need them. Lifesaving catheters are sometimes unavailable for people with multiple sclerosis who have bladder infections. There's little public awareness that MS even exists. It's like things were in the U.S. fifty years ago." MS societies in developed nations have adopted societies in emerging nations, mostly in Eastern Europe, to help accelerate the growth of the MS organizations there.

Enormous challenges lie ahead for the International Federation (renamed the Multiple Sclerosis International Federation in 2001) and its member societies. Nevertheless the Board of Directors of the National Multiple Sclerosis Society in the United States knows that its original $100,000 seed money grant was well spent. Millions of people with MS and their families worldwide have been helped, directly or indirectly, by the International Federation. Many doctors around the world were initially skeptical of any health agency run by lay volunteers with a medical and scientific advisory board. Historically, international health agencies had been run by physicians (although some of these organizations didn't get far off the ground). An organizational structure built around volunteer lay persons and physicians has always been a requirement for membership in the International Federation—and over the years it has gradually won praise from physicians everywhere. An official responsible for health agencies at the World Health Organization has classified the Federation as a model international voluntary health organization, whose bylaws are distributed by WHO to existing and emerging health agencies for consideration.

Sylvia believed the IFMSS reflected the philosophy of former presidential candidate Wendell Willkie who promoted international cooperation and the concept of "one world." "Differences in cultural, ethnic, religious, and political backgrounds have been largely overcome in dealing with the common problem of MS," she noted.

Volunteers who form the backbone of the International Federation are honored through the James D. Wolfensohn Award, which is a travel grant given to an individual with MS so that he or she can attend the Federation's biennial conference. It recognizes the recipient's valuable contributions to the fight against MS. David Pearse, from the MS Society of Great Britain and Northern Ireland, typified the high caliber of the winners of the Wolfensohn Award. Pearse was diagnosed with MS at the age of forty-four, after enjoying success in a career in information technology. An active volunteer in the MS movement at the local, national, and international levels, Pearse played a major role in setting up the World of Multiple Sclerosis, the Federation's Internet project. He was awarded the prize in 1996.

Thousands of people worldwide like David Pearse have been touched by multiple sclerosis and have made the commitment of time, energy, and money to fighting the disease. Many are motivated because a loved one has been afflicted with the illness. David Torrey was a prominent Canadian banker when his daughter was diagnosed with MS. He served as president of the Canadian MS Society, leading it to a position as one of the premier health agencies in Canada. He became a powerful force in the global MS movement, serving as senior vice president of the International Federation.

A twenty-fifth anniversary videotape described the Federation's many accomplishments and the future that awaited it.

There are now millions of people worldwide with MS. Two hundred thousand volunteers work to support 2,500 patient-care programs and 700 research projects, with the help of 450 fundraising events each year. The annual cost of the illness is in the billions of dollars.

The actor Daniel J. Travanti, whose brother has multiple sclerosis, narrated the commemorative videotape. Travanti, who once was the National MS Society's national campaign chairman, urged volunteers in every corner of the world to put the strength of their numbers to work. "We have it in our power to make MS powerless," he said.

34

IT WAS a simple concept. Dust off the bicycle stored in the garage for years, collect pledges from friends and families, and pedal a few miles for multiple sclerosis. By the end of the event, participants would feel healthier, and the multiple sclerosis movement would be better off because of their efforts.

That was the idea behind the MS Bike Tour which began on a small scale in 1980. It became one of the most successful fundraising campaigns of the National Multiple Sclerosis Society. "There are a lot of bicyclists in the country—a lot more than we knew when we started," said Thor Hanson. "The Bike Tour turned into a great vehicle to raise money. At the same time, we found that when people rode as part of the MS Bike Tour, they learned a lot more about multiple sclerosis than they had known before."

By the end of the 1980s the MS Bike Tour had pedaled to record accomplishments. In 1989 alone there were more than 90 tours nationwide, and the 55,000 participating cyclists raised $15.3 million. By 2000 the number had soared to $32 million under the leadership of Hanson's successor, General

Mike Dugan. Some volunteers, in fact, just couldn't get enough of it. In 1992 a cyclist named Mike Rose, an employee of Anadarko Petroleum, single-handedly raised $25,000 for multiple sclerosis. By the end of the decade, Peter Herschend of Bromson, Maryland, had raised more than $70,000 per year over several years.

Ed Chasteen was another National Society volunteer for whom cycling became a passion, propelling him far beyond the Bike Tour. In 1989, eight years after being diagnosed with multiple sclerosis, the fifty-three-year-old sociology professor at William Jewell College in Missouri was profiled in *Inside MS*. Chasteen recalled that for the first three years after the diagnosis he endured severe depression and would spend hours sitting quietly in his garage, where his son's bicycle had been stored. After staring at that bike for many weeks, he climbed aboard it one day and rode it for a block, which was as far as he could go. Three years later, however, his bike rides had become almost a daily occurrence. He began cycling to raise money for the MS movement—but the Bike Tour wasn't enough to quench his desire to help. He took a seemingly impossible ride—from one end of America to the other—making people with MS the beneficiaries of his effort. To prepare for the transcontinental feat, he trained by riding at least twenty miles a day, describing himself as whole and complete while he was cycling.

At the time of the first MS Bike Tour in 1980, many doctors were still cautioning their patients with multiple sclerosis that physical activity could exacerbate the disease. By the end of the 1980s, however, most physicians were communicating a far different message: Exercise is physically (and mentally) beneficial when pursued with common sense and the guidance of a health-care professional.

Cycling, according to Chasteen, gave him a sense of mastery over MS. "Medically, I'm not sure what the process is, but I know that when I exercise I feel 100 percent," he said. "If I skip a day for some reason, physically I am less able."

Once exercise was identified as a wholesome activity for people with multiple sclerosis, it was inevitable that an organized walk would join the Bike Tour as another way to raise money and focus national attention on the movement. The MS Walk grew out of a small fundraiser sponsored by the Minneapolis chapter. When Hanson heard about it, he immediately saw its potential as a national fundraiser—something that all chapters could sponsor on the same weekend each year. "I thought it would help give us a national presence and focus public attention on our cause while raising money," he said.

A special task force began planning a nationwide launch of the MS Walk in 1989. Forty-two chapters and branches participated that first year, with the goal of bringing every chapter into the fold within two years. Some people walked in teams; others walked alone. The courses ranged from three to nine miles. Many people with MS participated in the event—some used walkers, others wheelchairs. Many participants without MS walked on behalf of "Solemates"—friends and family members with multiple sclerosis. Major corporations such as Canada Dry and the Miller Brewing Company helped sponsor the Walk.

In 1990 eighty chapters participated in the Walk, raising $14 million, a 200 percent increase over the 1989 walk. That annual figure climbed to $33 million by 2000. By then hundreds of thousands of National Society supporters had walked many millions of miles—all of them carrying people with multiple sclerosis in their "hearts and soles." Each stride taken brought the world a step closer to finding the answer to this puzzling disease, and made MS-related services a little more available to people who desperately needed them.

With this success in mind, Thor Hanson approached the national board with the concept of renewing the Society's efforts for a national direct-mail campaign. It would be a way of reaching people in their homes, including other people with MS, while raising new money and educating the public about the disease. To his surprise, however, the board reacted coolly to the idea, some members noting that an earlier direct-mail effort had been too expensive. The chapters too responded reluctantly.

"I really believed that we ought to move into direct mail," said Hanson. "I explained to the chapter leaders that they would benefit. We would be taking the risk at the national level, since we would be footing the bill for the campaign. We'd give them 40 percent of whatever funds the program brought in, and we'd keep 60 percent."

Hanson finally persuaded the national board and the chapters to try the program. Not long after its launch in 1984, it generated sixty thousand new donors. In 1986 alone it collected $1.6 million.

On the research front, President Clifford Goldsmith proposed staging a Society-sponsored, day-long conference under the auspices of the National Academy of Sciences in Washington, D.C., attended by representatives from voluntary health organizations in other fields to brainstorm about better ways for the National MS Society to stimulate research. "By turning to expertise outside our own Society, our hope was to find out what they were doing and to get a sense of whether there were paths we should be following to get 'more bang for the buck,'" said Hanson.

The Washington conference was held in 1987. As an outgrowth of that event, the National MS Society began funding pilot research grants. They were relatively small ($20,000 to $25,000 for a one-year grant) but provided investigators with sufficient research funds to determine whether their high-risk, potentially high-payoff ideas merited full-scale studies. The Society also began funding early research into the psycho-social aspects of MS, which led to more intensive studies examining the value of cognitive retraining and rehabilitation for memory problems associated with the disease. After the Washington conference, researchers also began looking at ways to strengthen efforts to manage and deliver care more effectively. In more recent years the Society has taken steps to ensure that people with MS receive safe and adequate medical services in managed-care systems, and has urged the passage of patient-protection legislation.

"The 1987 conference was really a watershed event for us," said Hanson. "We continued to fund many of our grants as we had before, but we received a lot of additional ideas that we were able to implement."

By the end of the decade, scientists felt they had a better understanding of the activity of white blood cells and how they fight invading agents such as viruses, which some investigators believed might contribute to the development of multiple sclerosis. Several studies suggested that white blood cells mistakenly attack myelin as though they are waging war against foreign substances—a process that could play a crucial role in myelin damage. There were also some disappointing findings in clinical trials that evaluated new medications. At UCLA, a three-year study of the immunosuppressive drug azathioprine found no differences in the rate of MS progression between people taking the drug and those taking a placebo. Harvard researchers reported beneficial effects associated with another immunosuppressant, cyclophosphamide, but they turned out to be temporary. Patients who responded initially began to get worse shortly after treatment. Even so, some doctors reported finding value in using these drugs in certain patients.

There was also more encouraging news. Human clinical trials ultimately led to FDA approval of the first medications effective for changing the course of multiple sclerosis. By the 1990s, those studies had given people with MS their first real weapons against the progression of the disease. A team of investigators at the Cleveland Clinic would later describe the decade of the 1980s as a turning point in the war on multiple sclerosis, noting that for most of the twentieth century "MS was considered untreatable." In their 1997 article in the *New England Journal of Medicine*, they pointed to an international workshop on therapeutic trials in the 1980s, co-sponsored by the National MS Society, as forever changing the mind-set of investigators. "The workshop served to usher in an era of activism and optimism that has substantially replaced widespread therapeutic nihilism and skepticism about the feasibility of clinical trials in multiple sclerosis."

There was a feeling that the answers to MS were finally within reach. As research efforts accelerated, Sylvia Lawry's early support for multiple sclerosis research was never forgotten by the National Society. At a banquet at the Society's 1986 National Leadership Conference—the fortieth anniversary of the Society—Norman Cohn announced the creation of the Sylvia Lawry Fund for Multiple Sclerosis Research as a tribute to her decades of inspiring leadership. Colleagues, friends, and admirers contributed $107,000 in seed money for the Lawry research fund. The following year, no one was surprised when

Ronald Reagan presented Sylvia with the President's Volunteer Action Award at the White House.

Other presidents have been quick to honor those who have struggled against multiple sclerosis. In 1989, George Bush invited the MS Mother and Father of the Year to the White House—an annual tradition that launches the Society's national fundraising drive. At age fifty, Sheila Ann Olsen, a mother of ten, had been fighting MS for twenty-two years. Although she used a wheelchair, she could proudly say that she had always attended every one of her children's activities, from band concerts to ball games. She also served on the board of directors of an organization serving the disabled, and had been the Republican state co-chairperson in two congressional campaigns. She was quite deserving of the White House accolades.

At the same ceremony, Steve Adams was honored as Father of the Year. He had been diagnosed in 1982 at the age of forty, and wore a leg brace to the White House event. Though he worked as vice president of a company, he still found plenty of time for involvement in the lives of his three children. He and his sons collected more money than anyone else for a 1988 "Longest Day of Golf" fundraiser to fight MS. Steve also led support groups at his local MS chapter and frequently spoke at Society workshops.

Perhaps no National Society program has exemplified the power of the human spirit better than Project Rembrandt. Launched in 1983, it displayed in the halls of the National office the art works of persons with MS. It was a way to demonstrate the talent, creativity, and courage that persisted—and even thrived—among these individuals, despite their disease. Painters, sculptors, potters, and photographers with multiple sclerosis placed their works on display. The reaction was so positive that the project quickly outgrew the hallways of the National Society's headquarters. "The quality of the art and the spirit of the artists challenged us to make something more of this program," said Hanson. The Society formed a National Volunteer Project Rembrandt Committee that shaped and expanded the program, and turned it into a juried exhibition. It appeared at galleries such as the IBM Gallery of Sciences and Art in New York, and beginning in 1988 it toured the country with the help of corporate sponsorship.

The 1991 Project Rembrandt exhibition, titled "Against the Odds," opened at the MetLife Gallery in New York City. Six hundred people attended the preview reception, including luminaries from the corporate, artistic, and show business worlds. The honored guests were the seventeen participating artists, one of whom was Leah Finch. At age twenty-two, Leah was diagnosed with multiple sclerosis. Before the disease struck, she had been a painter, but MS robbed her of this pursuit. She enrolled in a class in ceramic sculpture, which became her new avenue of expression. Leah said, "Having multiple sclerosis can make a determined person very creative. To me the real meaning behind Project Rembrandt is how each artist is able to use his or her mind to adapt and continue when the body becomes difficult. Anyone with MS knows the process I am talking about. This program inspires me not just as an artist. It's a symbol of other people like me who have multiple sclerosis, and who adapt their abilities and continue to work."

When Tom Martin's MS prevented him from standing in front of an easel, he stopped painting on large canvases and switched to smaller, more conceptual works of art. Amy Wexler had been a photographer when MS gradually deprived her of her ability to see color. She changed her focus and began concentrating on black-and-white photography, which she found to be an unexplored but rewarding artistic medium. Bess Bonner had been a medical illustrator, but when MS ended her career she started painting with a brush in a mouth holder.

By the 1990s each of the biennial shows—now called "The Creative Will"—was viewed by approximately a quarter of a million people nationwide. The underlying message: Disability is not synonymous with inability.

35

IN 1989, National Society chairman George Gillespie, III, partner in the law firm of Cravath Swaine & Moore, looked back on the decade and pointed with pride to the ways in which the Society had helped improve the lives of people with MS. The Society's fundraising success had more than doubled, from $30 million collected in 1980 to $78 million in 1989. All of the funds had been raised with the goal of improving the well-being of individuals with MS as well as expanding research efforts.

Nevertheless Gillespie acknowledged what all of his predecessors had to concede: multiple sclerosis remained a tough and unconquered enemy. "Our greatest disappointment during the past ten years has been our failure to unlock the secret of multiple sclerosis," Gillespie said. "Not that we haven't tried. Though the pace of scientific and medical research into MS has accelerated more quickly than ever before, concrete results have remained elusive, just beyond our grasp."

As the 1990s began, not a single approved treatment for multiple sclerosis addressed the underlying cause of the disease. Most doctors simply told their patients, "We can help you manage your MS symptoms, but we have nothing for your disease."

All that changed, however, in the early 1990s. After decades of frustration and tens of thousands of hours of laboratory research and meticulous clinical trials, a dramatic breakthrough emerged from the biotechnology revolution. It offered a treatment of the disease itself, not just its symptoms.

It came in the form of a drug called interferon beta-1b, a genetically engineered variant of a molecule naturally produced by the body's own immune system. It was approved by the FDA for relapsing-remitting MS in 1993 under the brand name Betaseron. Taken every other day through a subcutaneous (just under the skin), self-administered injection, Betaseron proved in clinical trials that the medication could alter the course of the disease. In one large study, people with MS experienced a 34 percent decrease in relapses while taking interferon beta-1b along with a reduction in the severity of the relapses, and a decline in the accumulation of new lesions in the brain (as measured by MRIs). From the earliest days of the experimental use of interferons, the Society provided significant funding for this cutting-edge research.

As one study after another confirmed the promise of interferon beta-1b, the National MS Society's leadership decided not to leave the drug's approval to chance. The Society lobbied in Washington, organized testimony by experts before Food and Drug Administration panels, and asked its members to participate in aggressive letter-writing and telephone campaigns. As a result, just four months after the FDA's expert advisory committee on new drugs recommended the approval of Betaseron, the FDA formally sanctioned its marketing.

When the drug was approved, the mood among many MS

families changed, and the public perception of multiple sclerosis shifted. MS was no longer seen as an untreatable disease.
There was now reason for hope. A Society member in Colorado
said, "The nurse who taught me how to inject myself had no
idea what this new drug means to me. The hope that MS can
be controlled—even a little—it's an overwhelming feeling."
After a New York City Society member began taking Betaseron,
she publicly announced, "This year I'm back at work, and last
year I was too ill."

As exciting as Betaseron was, its introduction was far from
trouble-free. Within two months of FDA approval, the pharmaceutical company that manufactured the drug could not keep
up with the enormous demand for it. To compound the problem of product shortage, its high cost blocked access for many
people with MS, particularly those whose health insurance did
not adequately cover the costs of the medication. The retail
price was staggering—in excess of $10,000 a year—which was
beyond the reach of many of the individuals who needed the
drug.

The FDA also approved the marketing of two other breakthrough prescription drugs for MS:

In 1996, Avonex (interferon beta-1a) became the second
drug approved for altering the course of MS. It was another injected drug, requiring weekly doses, with a deeper insertion
of the needle into muscle tissue. A double-blind, placebo-
controlled study at five MS treatment facilities showed that
Avonex reduced by 37 percent the risk of further physical disability or impairment over two years, plus a 32 percent decline
in the incidence of acute flare-ups or exacerbations and a decrease in new brain lesions.

Copaxone (copolymer-1 or glatiramer acetate), approved
in 1996, is administered daily with a subcutaneous injection. It

is capable of reducing the frequency of relapses. One major study showed a 29 percent decline in the relapse rate.

As with Betaseron, investigators conducting research into Avonex and Copaxone received support from the National Society. Studies have recently showed the comparable effects of all three drugs, including the ability to reduce the frequency and severity of relapses and an early indication of slowing the progression of disability. In the process these drugs have improved the quality of life for many people with MS. Nevertheless, by 1998 only 18 percent of persons who could benefit from the drugs were taking them, in part because of the cost, in part because of physician inertia, but also because some people became discouraged by the need to administer medication by injection, or by the possibility of side effects.

In 1998 the National MS Society issued an advisory statement about the new medications: "The evidence is quite clear for benefit in relapsing-remitting disease, while the value in progressive forms has not yet been demonstrated, and is currently being studied." Then, in late 1998, the British journal *The Lancet* published a large European study of Betaseron, showing benefits in people with secondary-progressive MS (a condition that begins as relapsing-remitting disease but then progresses and steadily grows worse). Other studies presented that same year at a major MS conference indicated that the permanent nerve-fiber injury associated with MS may be more aggressive in the disease's early stages than was previously believed, suggesting the advisability of using one of the new trio of drugs as early in the disease process as possible.

Research findings like these led the Society to break with precedent and recommend use of the new pharmaceutical agents "as soon as possible following a definitive diagnosis of MS and determination of a relapsing course. . . . Therapy is to be continued indefinitely, unless there is clear lack of benefit, intolerable side effects, new data which reveal other reasons for cessation, or better therapy is available."

Nancy Law, vice president for client programs for the National MS Society, advised persons with the disease that it was more important than ever for them to look out for their own medical interests when it came to these medications. "People always have had responsibility for their own care," she told *Inside MS* in 1999. "But now this job is more urgent than ever. Today, early treatment can make a long-term difference. These new drugs do work. This development means people with MS need to move more quickly out of the comfort zone of denial and face up to what can really happen with MS over the coming years."

As important as the new medications are, none is the perfect drug. They cannot reverse existing disability, and at the present time they are approved only for some people with MS. They are not a cure for the disease. Dr. Stanley van den Noort, chief medical officer of the National MS Society, confirmed that the three medications not only work well in moderating the course of the disease but that "research is now exploring the possibility of combining the drugs in ways that may prove even more effective." The evidence of the efficacy of these medications has become so strong that the National Society has felt compelled to issue a formal recommendation to physicians, advising their use.

Mike Dugan explained it this way to people with MS: "These new drugs can slow down the ability of MS to rob people of their functions. If one of them is right for you, the sooner you start, the better you will do, and the longer you may be able to go without losing significant abilities, like the use of legs or hands. So, subject to an individual physician's best judgment of a particular patient, since people are unique and so is MS, we recommend using one of them—now."

On other research fronts, the National Society announced its support of a comprehensive search for the genes that make people susceptible to multiple sclerosis. Although MS is not hereditary, a first-degree relative (that is, a parent or sibling) increases the risk of developing the disease, compared to the population at large. Some neurologists believe that MS may occur because an individual is born with a genetic predisposition to react to an environmental substance that induces an autoimmune response. In 1999, Dr. W. Ian McDonald, chairman of the International Medical Advisory Board of the International Federation, said, "We now know that there are a number of genes involved in MS, not just one. And we know where some of these genes are likely to be located, such as the sixth chromosome where the genetic control of the immune system lies."

Stephen Reingold, vice president of research programs for the National MS Society, believes that genetic research may lead to a way to predict who will contract MS, allowing medical interventions at the earliest possible stages with treatments that could influence the course of the disease. And with the information about the genetic foundation of MS in hand, scientists may someday be able to manipulate and perhaps "correct" problematic genes.

In the 1990s the Society also continued to fund research aimed at better understanding the specific activity of the immune system in the disease, with the hope of developing effective immunotherapies. Other scientists explored the genetic and molecular underpinnings of myelin, and whether functional remyelination can someday occur and thus allow recovery from MS. The FDA also approved the marketing of

Zanaflex for muscle spasticity, a common MS symptom—the first new oral treatment for spasticity to reach the U.S. market in more than twenty years.

This kind of research understandably boosted the hopes of MS families. As a way of honoring the leading scientists dedicated to the study of multiple sclerosis, in 1993 the National Society announced the establishment of the John Dystel Prize for Multiple Sclerosis Research. The annual $7,500 prize, given jointly by the Society and the American Academy of Neurology, is a professional award devoted exclusively to MS research, recognizing significant contributions in the field. It is funded through the John Dystel Multiple Sclerosis Research Fund at the Society. The fund was established by Oscar Dystel, John's father. John, a Yale Law School graduate, found his promising legal career shortened by the progressive disability associated with MS. He had been a champion figure skater but developed his first MS symptoms while at Yale. Yet he pursued a law career for as long as possible, becoming a founding partner of a firm in Seattle, working in the U.S. Department of Education, and serving as a lobbyist for the American Coalition of Citizens with Disabilities. When the Dystel Prize was established, Oscar Dystel said that it "was our family's way to say thank you for the advances dedicated researchers are making toward a cure." Donations to the John Dystel Fund, which exceeded $500,000 by 1999, have come from John's former classmates at Brown and Yale, other friends, family, and members of the publishing industry where Oscar Dystel has been a prominent executive for decades.

Since its creation, the Dystel Prize has honored researchers such as neurologist Donald Paty of the University of British Columbia, whose studies on the use of MRIs in multiple sclerosis have provided new insights into the disease. Other

winners have included epidemiologist John Kurtzke of Georgetown University School of Medicine, who developed an expanded and refined MS disability status scale (sometimes
called the Kurtzke Scale) that played a key role in determining
the effectiveness of the new drugs approved in the 1990s; neuroscientist Cedric Raine of Albert Einstein College of Medicine, whose research has led to the current understanding that
the myelin sheath is the primary target of attacks by the body's
immune system; neurologist Henry McFarland of the National
Institute of Neurological Disorders and Stroke, who was among
the first investigators to emphasize the influence of genetic
factors on an individual's susceptibility to MS; W. Ian
McDonald, chairman of the International Federation's International Medical Advisory Board, who was the first researcher
to show that the loss of myelin impairs the ability of nerve impulses to continue across a demyelinated portion of a nerve
fiber; and Kenneth Johnson, who was recognized for his international leadership in designing and conducting controlled,
multi-center clinical trials testing medications for MS.

"The Dystel Prize helps focus attention on significant advances in our field and brings issues in MS research to the attention of a wider community of clinicians and investigators in
related fields," said Dr. Reingold of the National MS Society.

A parallel prize, the Charcot Award, is awarded by the International Federation once every two years and is named after
Jean Martin Charcot, the nineteenth-century French neurologist who provided the first detailed description of multiple sclerosis. It is given for lifetime achievement in research that
contributes to the understanding and treatment of MS. Winners of the award have come from throughout the world
and include Americans Byron Waksman, Richard Johnson, Leonard Kurland, and John Kurtzke; Germany's Helmut

Bauer, Great Britain's W. Ian McDonald and Douglas Mc-
Alpine, Canada's Donald Paty, and Japan's Yoshigoro Kuroiwa.
Research by Bauer on children with MS has captured much attention; he found that the first symptoms of MS can occur in
childhood, though it often goes undiagnosed. The disease
moves into remission, only to reemerge in young adulthood.

The successes by investigators such as these—and even the
disappointments along the way—reinforce the importance of
continuing to emphasize the funding of research, which began
with the Society's very first grant in 1947. Today the process for
awarding research dollars is more sophisticated and competitive. Every grant proposal is evaluated by the volunteer members of the Society's peer review committee. Half the proposals
never make it through this rigorous evaluation process. Only
the most promising applications ultimately receive funding. Although the federal government's appropriations for MS research consistently exceed those of the Society, Sylvia Lawry
called the organization's research support "the seed money
that gets the fires lit in places where interest did not previously
exist and where progress is already being made. I think the
level of government support is directly related to our own level
of research support."

Although progress in research has been encouraging, it
still has not ended the frustration that MS families often feel. "I
would like to see the Society find the answer to multiple sclerosis, and there are indications that we're getting closer," says
Chairman Emeritus L. Palmer Brown. "I sometimes get impa-
tient with the pace of research. But then I go to a meeting of
MS researchers and I realize that we're doing all that can be
done."

36

IN THE EARLY 1990s, Thor Hanson began planning his retirement. Although his commitment to the Society had not waned, he felt it was time to give more attention to his family. The National Society began a search for new leadership—a pursuit that again led to a retired senior military officer. General Mike Dugan had been the air force's chief of staff and top-ranking officer. Upon his retirement in 1991 he became a consultant with CBS News and a lecturer in strategic studies at the Paul H. Nitze School of Advanced International Studies at Johns Hopkins University. Dugan was a graduate of West Point, had flown more than three hundred combat missions in Vietnam, and had been commander-in-chief of the U.S. air forces in Europe and commander of NATO's allied air forces in Central Europe before being appointed chief of staff. General Dugan became a primary proponent of an air campaign against Iraq.

When he departed the military, Dugan began looking for a second career that would steer him away from defense and aerospace and into a position in which he might again head a significant cause. He received a cold call from a recruiting firm, explaining that a search was under way for a new leader for the National Society. "I had never heard of the National Multiple Sclerosis Society, though I did know something about MS," said Dugan. His brother-in-law had been diagnosed with multiple sclerosis fourteen years earlier, and as the disease progressed, Dugan had seen its physical and emotional toll on the family. "I understood some of the impact that this disease can have, and when I asked my brother-in-law what kind of reputation the National Society had, and whether it was helpful to him and his family, he had very positive things to say."

When Dugan was formally offered the position, he accepted the challenge, saying it was "a worthy, socially responsible job." In June 1992, as he assumed the titles of president and CEO, he immediately visited chapters and research labs and talked to many people with MS and their families. He met with staff members at the national office and at the recently opened Training and Resource Center in Denver, and he spoke with donors. He identified areas where the Society was doing well and where it needed improvement. "One of my goals was to get the organization to think of itself as more of a whole, rather than individual pieces," he said. Toward that end he created a management team of twenty-five chapter leaders who began meeting about every three months. Dugan arrived at each of these sessions with an agenda of five or six problems that the Society faced, and the group brainstormed possible solutions.

When Dugan assumed leadership of the Society, several issues needed immediate attention. In light of the sluggish national economy in the early 1990s, revenues received at the national office had stagnated. The Society was able to avoid a deficit by trimming expenditures in virtually all areas except research. Dugan took a hard look at the organization's fundraising and began to refocus it. Up to that point, the chapters tended to raise whatever money they could, then allocate what they had for their many worthwhile programs. Dugan became convinced that the Society should position its mission programs front and center, and with them in mind, gear up to raise the funds necessary to fulfill those missions.

Dugan also believed that the Society needed to broaden its sources of income and reduce its relative emphasis on special events to raise money. "These events are usually outdoors, subject to the whims of the weather and the marketplace, and they're fairly high-cost compared to traditional fundraising," he said. "We're producing events like walks and bike rides, and the focus is more on the activity, on the fun, rather than on the need to improve the quality of life of people with MS through participation. The 'good cause' is almost secondary to the event. I felt we should begin to direct more of our attention to programs such as planned giving and direct mail."

By 1993 the Society's major special events—the MS Walk and the Bike Tour—had actually experienced declines in their fundraising success, but these decreases were offset by growth in other areas, including million-dollar increases in both direct-mail fundraising and the annual campaign. Under Dugan's leadership, the Society's income has consistently grown. "Initially, some people were concerned about how well a general would do in running a voluntary health agency," said Sylvia Lawry. "But General Dugan has impressed a lot of people here. He is committed to what he's doing, and he has taken this on as his life's challenge. He has been able to call upon his experience of working in organizations in the military by applying advanced technology and discipline in management. He has been very effective in many areas."

With the approval of the three new MS drugs in the 1990s, Dugan sensed a strengthened optimism throughout the organization. "The drugs we have are not a cure," he said. "But their development and approval has carried the message that if we work hard enough at this, we'll uncover the mechanisms behind MS, ways to deal with the workings of the immune system, and we'll finally be able to control this disease. There are many MS clinical trials now being funded by pharmaceutical companies, run by business people who are very analytical about where to invest their research dollars. And the fact that they're turning more attention to multiple sclerosis suggests that they believe that something good could happen soon in MS."

As Dugan learned more about the disease, he developed a stronger respect for his brother-in-law who had lived with MS for years. "He has had a significant downturn in his health and developed severe spasticity in his right arm and overwhelming fatigue," Dugan said recently. "He has been in a wheelchair for quite a while now. He's a lot tougher guy than I once gave him credit for. I think a lot of him."

37

ALTHOUGH multiple sclerosis can pose many challenges, people with the disease tend to find ways to surmount them as best they can. Robie Pierce was diagnosed with MS in 1985 but refused to give up his love of sailing. In 1993 he and his two-person crew won the World Disabled Sailing Championship, competing against nineteen entrants from eleven countries. Pierce used a wheelchair while sailing; his crew member Nick Bryan-Brown had been diagnosed with MS in 1990, and the third person on their team, Rusty Sargent, was a paraplegic. "Our boat is not specially adapted because we are disabled—each crew member had to improvise based on his own particular disabilities," said Pierce. "Continuing my sailing has enabled me to move beyond my disabilities and focus on my abilities—it has given me the confidence that there is life after the wheelchair."

Rolande Cutner, a French attorney in her sixties, is another person with multiple sclerosis who has not let the disease put a damper on her own athletic endeavors. When she's not practicing law in Paris and New York, she volunteers as a board member of the MS Society in France—and skydives to attract public attention to the disease. At an MS-sponsored event in Paris, she parachuted from a plane, performing acrobatics in the air with a team of other parachutists. She saw it as a way of demonstrating that persons with MS need not feel limitations on what they can do.

Courage also has been shown by Annette Funicello. Annette was the prototypical all-American kid and one of the most popular of Walt Disney's Mouseketeers. Even as an adult, she seemed to be leading a charmed life, which she described as "consumed by carpooling, Little League games, and the other routine activities of your typical mom, including making peanut butter sandwiches."

But Annette realized that something was wrong the day she had trouble focusing her eyes while reading a script. She also developed occasional tingling sensations in her feet, and sometimes she had problems with her equilibrium. Years passed before doctors finally diagnosed her condition as MS. When she finally went public with her condition in 1992, it quieted rumors that her poor sense of balance was caused by alcoholism. By that time she had lost her ability to walk without assistance.

Annette became an honorary spokesperson for the National Society and officially led the MS Walk in 1992. "I have a recurring dream that one day I rise from a chair and start walking," she wrote in her autobiography. "I can hear my kids saying, 'Mom, look at you! You don't even have your cane!' And then I stop and realize that I really am walking again. 'You're right!' I say in the dream. 'I am walking!' And someday that dream, that wish, may come true."

Because Annette is such a recognizable personality, she

has helped peel back some of the mystery and fear surrounding MS, and has made it easier for people with the disease to confront their illness. When James Rea was diagnosed with MS, it became more of an inconvenience than an obstacle in his life. He needed to use a cane, crutches, or a scooter at times, but his own physical challenges only prompted him to do something for others with disabilities—namely children. He established and coached the first baseball and soccer teams for youngsters with disabilities in his hometown of Sunnyvale, California. In 1996, when he visited the White House with his own two teenagers to accept the Society's Father of the Year Award from President Clinton, he could point with pride to his volunteer work with the local chapter of the National MS Society. He also wrote a booklet called *The Three-Minute Guide to MS*, to help his friends and family understand how MS affects people's day-to-day lives. In that booklet he wrote that "most disabilities are in the minds of the able-bodied, not the bodies of the disabled."

And how did James Rea advise adjusting to a life with MS? "Develop your sense of humor," he said.

For the families of persons with MS, it takes courage to support their affected loved one, providing care and fighting back against a seemingly relentless disease. Reid Nicholson, an activist in the MS Society in Canada and in the International Federation, learned firsthand the intolerance of some segments of society toward the chronically ill. He was discharged from the Canadian navy when his superiors learned that he had MS, even though he showed no signs of disability. As well as battling for the rights of people with MS, he and his wife, Evie, devised an award given at each International Federation conference. Called the International Caregiver of the Year—

the Nicholson Award—it is given to the spouse, relative, friend, or caregiver who has demonstrated commitment and support to make life better for their loved one with MS.

Multiple sclerosis is particularly tough on children who must often take on the responsibilities of helping care for a mother or father with the disease, at an age when most of their friends are concerned with just being kids. More than one million children in the United States have MS in their immediate families. To provide them with a venue for expressing their own experiences with the disease, in 1996 the Society launched a nationwide project called Through the Eyes of a Child. It encourages children (ages five through sixteen) to express themselves artistically in reflecting on how their lives have been affected by MS.

In the first year of Through the Eyes of a Child, ninety works of art were displayed, initially in Atlanta as part of the Society's National Leadership Conference, and then in 12 states where it was eventually viewed by more than 350,000 people. The 1998–1999 exhibit contained more than 160 pieces—paintings, sculptures, and photographs—that were displayed in seven major museums, two state legislatures, three medical centers, three corporate headquarters, and five shopping malls. In just two of these venues—the Riverfront Art Center in Delaware and the State Museum in Raleigh—more than one million visitors viewed the exhibit. The drama and poignancy of these works of art brought many people to tears.

38

IN 1996 the National MS Society marked its fiftieth year of service to individuals with multiple sclerosis and their families. It was a time for commemoration and reflection. The Society's members and volunteers exceeded half a million people, and life was better for most MS families because of the services and the research supported by the organization. The pioneers of the Society, including Sylvia Lawry, believed that all of the answers to MS would have been uncovered long before its golden anniversary. But there were still many reasons to feel proud, and to honor Sylvia and others for their contributions.

The year before the fiftieth anniversary, the Society rephrased its mission statement. It is clear and concise: To end the devastating effects of multiple sclerosis.

It had been the dream from the beginning, but it had never been stated so simply. The Society proclaimed November 19, 1996, as Founder's Day, honoring Sylvia Lawry, her vision of a world free of MS, and all she had accomplished in striving toward that goal. That same year the Women's International Center (WIC) presented Sylvia with its Living Legacy Award. It described her as "a woman whose legacy began fifty years ago and will continue for generations."

In a letter to the WIC, longtime National board member Thacher Longstreth praised Sylvia and recalled the first time their paths had crossed. "Almost immediately," he wrote, "it was clear to me that Sylvia Lawry possessed an amazing energy and a personal vision unequaled in anyone I had met thus far in my lifetime. Her passion was helping others, and she was determined through sheer force of will, strength of character, personal integrity and dedication to do just that. . . . I have seen time and time again Sylvia's unselfish dedication to others and her ability to turn adversity into strength."

Neuroscientist Cedric Raine of the Albert Einstein College of Medicine described the impact that Sylvia had made on him and on the entire scientific community. "Sylvia's constant interest and encouragement during my formative years had great influence on my development. Through her belief in me and scientists like me, we have been able to advance dramatically the understanding and treatment of MS and train a cadre of disciples to do likewise around the world. She has never sought personal aggrandizement. Her commitment has always been to people with multiple sclerosis and those who serve them. After a half-century of such dedication, I believe the time has come to recognize Sylvia not only for establishing multiple sclerosis as a research discipline but for founding and furthering a worldwide organization that helps millions of people each year."

Families who lived with MS a half-century earlier fought their battles alone, with nowhere to turn for information, support, and treatment. Today Society chapters in every part of the nation provide expanding services and programs. In chapter support groups, people with MS can share their successes and concerns about living with the disease. These groups are led by professional therapists and/or trained peer counselors. Crisis intervention personnel offer emergency counseling. Medical transportation and occupational, physical, and speech therapy are also provided. Local programs help the children and spouses of people with MS adjust to the changes in their own lives associated with the disease. As Judy Rahmani, the National Society's 1994 MS Mother of the Year, has said, "I feel better, not bitter, thanks to my local chapter."

Persons with MS have learned that despite their disease, they can lead meaningful and even active lives. Chapter rehabilitation programs provide classes in low-stress exercise, water therapy, and yoga. Adapted sports programs give people with MS the opportunity for horseback riding, sailing, bowling, and golf. Mary Tinker organizes outdoor recreational programs for the Colorado chapter. She joins other chapter members in camping, sailing, whitewater rafting, and skiing. Although she has relapsing-remitting MS and typically must walk with the aid of a cane, she participates in activities that she never took part in before her diagnosis. In 1998 she told *Inside MS*, "We're pooped at the end of the day. But it's a good kind of tired because we've had such a terrific time."

Trained peer counselors answer the Society's toll-free phone lines, which now ring in the chapter nearest the caller. These counselors spend hours each day listening and talking to people with MS and their families about their lives and their concerns about the future. In 1998 alone, more than 350,000 callers nationwide dialed 1-800-FIGHTMS.

Each spring the Society organizes a national teleconference, during which many thousands of people with MS assemble at one of six hundred sites in the country to learn about the latest developments in MS treatments and research. They use a network of special phone lines to exchange live questions and answers with nationally renowned experts. The 1999 conference was titled "It's Your Call: Making Treatment Decisions," and featured J. Jock Murray of Nova Scotia and other leading neurologists. This technology allows individuals to access state-of-the-art information about the disease, right in their own communities.

Most chapters also offer their own education programs where people newly diagnosed with MS can meet face to face with others who have the disease. Said Janie Brunette, a registered nurse with MS who chairs the Society's National Programs Advisory Council, "It's real comforting to see another person—in person—and know that they look good and that in many ways they're very similar to yourself."

On the Internet, the Society in 1999 produced a series of five live programs called "Moving Forward." They were interactive webcasts designed primarily for people recently diagnosed with MS, giving them an opportunity to listen to presentations by authorities in the field and send e-mailed questions that were answered by these experts via the Internet. Both the National MS Society and the International Federation have created their own websites to provide on-line information about MS that can be accessed twenty-four hours a day from anywhere in the world. The National Society's website (http://www.nationalmssociety.org) receives 150,000 visitors per month, and the International Federation's site (http://www.msif.org) hosts tens of thousands of visitors each month.

Throughout the 1990s, under the leadership of Thor Hanson and Mike Dugan, the National Society spearheaded pioneering legislation designed to support and empower all people who live with multiple sclerosis. As Dugan noted in 1998, every opportunity must be taken "to inform a sometimes disbelieving public that disability does not mean the same thing as inability. People can and must be considered qualified based on their actual qualifications."

Not too many years ago, individuals with MS accepted the fact that barriers kept them from participating fully in day-to-day life. Efforts by the Society's Action Alert program, which coordinates grassroots lobbying campaigns, helped change that. It pushed hard for congressional passage of the Americans with Disabilities Act, which became law in 1990 and extended civil rights protection to all people with disabilities. It has supported initiatives to expand employment opportunities for people with MS, and to increase federal funding for MS research. In 1998 alone, Society volunteers testified at fourteen congressional hearings in support of matters relevant to multiple sclerosis. In 2000 some two hundred MS advocates visited their representatives in Congress in Washington, D.C., to seek increased federal support for scientific investigations into the disease, and discuss issues bearing on insurance, medical and genetic privacy, and disability. More than 60 percent of the Society's chapters now have volunteer government relations committees, which are active in advocacy efforts on behalf of people with MS. Their aim is simple: to ensure that state and local agencies understand MS and the special needs of people who have it, and that adequate government funds are channeled into MS research. In this era of HMOs and managed care, people need to be prepared to stand up for themselves and for their own rights. In a 1999 article in *Inside MS,* Dr. Stanley van den Noort, chief medical officer of the National MS Society, said, "Even in managed care, if people are well informed and vocal—if they keep banging on the door—they will get what they want. It's the people who give up and go home or flit around from one doctor to another who get lost in the shuffle."

Anne Marie Riether, a psychiatrist who was diagnosed with MS in 1993, has been active in the Georgia chapter since then, participating in MS walks and bicycling events and speaking at a "Day in the Life of Women with MS" program. Perhaps her greatest contribution came in the aftermath of her participation in a clinical trial evaluating a T-cell receptor vaccine for MS, during which her symptoms improved. After the study, when her condition worsened, she was unable to use the vaccine because it had not been approved by the FDA. Dr. Riether joined forces with Dr. Karen Mullican, another person with MS who took part in the vaccine study. They worked with Newt Gingrich, then Speaker of the House, and contacted other congressmen and won support for "compassionate use" reform to permit individuals with a serious disease to use experimental drugs while FDA review and approval were ongoing. As a result, the FDA Modernization Act of 1997 was passed into law. In the wake of her advocacy campaign, Dr. Riether was named the recipient of the Society's 1998 National Achievement Award.

On other fronts, the National Society and its chapters distribute over two million copies of more than thirty booklets, brochures, and fact sheets about MS each year. This literature responds to the need for information by people with MS and their families, covering subjects like how the disease can be managed and how it affects lives at home and in the workplace. A special series, "Knowledge Is Power," is divided into ten sections, one of which is mailed every two weeks to a newly diagnosed person learning to adjust.

One of the most prolific authors on the National MS Society staff is Nancy J. Holland, R.N., Ed.D., who joined the Society in 1988, and has written more than sixty MS-related publications. They cover topics including rehabilitation, management of bladder and bowel dysfunction, and employment.

She is also senior author of *Multiple Sclerosis: A Guide for the Newly Diagnosed,* senior editor of *Multiple Sclerosis: A Self-Care Guide to Wellness,* and is currently the Society's vice president of the Clinical Programs Department.

On the local level, families like the Buegeleisens of Sarasota, Florida, have been pursuing their own avenues for raising research dollars. Alan Buegeleisen was twenty-seven years old and fiercely independent when he was diagnosed with MS. He had led an active life as a hiker and rock climber, and was studying forestry at the University of Massachusetts when the first symptoms of his disease surfaced. He continued to live on his own for several years, but finally his disease progressed to the point where he was forced to move in with his parents.

Alan's mother and father, Sally and Abbott, became caretakers of their adult son. But to ease some of their own emotional pain and frustration, they began sponsoring an annual MS gala in Sarasota that ultimately raised hundreds of thousands of dollars for the Society's local chapter. After ten years they shifted their efforts to raising money for the newly established Alan Buegeleisen MS Fund for Research. Through letters sent each year to friends and other contributors, the campaign now collects over $100,000 annually, which is spent solely on research into the disease.

"When we started all this, I asked Alan what he thought of the idea of raising money," said Sally, who is a member of the National Society's Board of Directors. "Alan said, 'You're going to help some people, and you're going to help to get over your frustration.' "

Through it all, Alan has kept his spirits up, despite his disability. "He never complains," said Sally. "When Alan was diagnosed, he said, 'You have to play the cards they deal you.'"

The efforts of the Buegeleisens and so many other families are aimed at contributing to the singular goal of an ultimate victory over multiple sclerosis. In 2000, the fifty-fourth anniversary year of the National Society, the organization's total income climbed to $158 million, including $83 million from special events and $75 million from traditional fundraising. This allowed record funds to be channeled into research, services, education, and advocacy; research alone totaled $28 million in 2000, funding new and continuing projects. It marked the fourth consecutive year that the Society was able to fund every MS project that had been approved by the organization's rigorous peer review. Research spending was projected to increase to $30 million in 2001, supporting more than 330 MS studies.

Researchers now believe that the damage to myelin results from all-out warfare within the body. It appears to involve an abnormal response by the immune system. For some reason it goes out of control in MS, misidentifying and destroying myelin. As nerve fibers in the spinal cord or brain lose sections of myelin, areas of scarring form hardened patches (lesions) that block the transmission of nerve impulses. The current consensus among scientists is that the damage in MS is related to inflammation, which is mediated by the immune system. But research is under way to determine if some lesions may be produced in other ways as well. There are also efforts at the Albert Einstein College of Medicine to study ways to promote the proliferation of cells called oligodendrocytes that make myelin. By administering a natural chemical (called glial growth factor 2) to mice with an MS-like disease (EAE), the severity of symptoms and relapse rates were reduced; this therapy also seemed to stimulate the repair of myelin in damaged regions of the animal's brain. These findings could lead to similar research in humans.

Researchers aren't yet certain what sets this disease process in motion, though they are closing in on answers. While MS is not directly inherited, there is clearly a genetic component. Studies indicate that MS is a "multigenic" disease, and the new tools of molecular biology have helped investigators identify a number of gene regions that seem to make an individual susceptible to MS. Genes, however, do not appear to be the sole factor that determines who will develop MS. A current popular theory is that individuals with a genetic predisposition to MS develop the disease after being exposed to an environmental "trigger," perhaps an infectious agent that causes the immune system to attack the body.

In addition to genetic studies, efforts will continue to identify the environmental factors that may play a role in MS. "Epidemiological evidence is quite good that there is something in the environment that plays a role in MS, and one theory is that it might induce MS in a genetically predisposed individual," said Dr. Ian McDonald of the International Federation. While he notes that there has not yet been a confirmed isolation of a virus or any other organism in MS, "I think this is one of the major areas where progress will be made in the years ahead."

Richard Snyder, whose sister Carol has MS, became chairman of the national board in January 1995. As he and the other Society leaders reflected upon the many accomplishments over the organization's five-decade history, he publicly reaffirmed his own strong resolve to defeat MS. Snyder told a national conference, "MS doesn't deserve to exist. We can say good things about how people cope. But there isn't one good thing to say about MS."

People have said many good things about the National MS Society, however. In 1999 a national survey conducted by Roper Starch International sought to determine how well the Society was responding to the needs of persons with the disease. When asked whether the organization was meeting their needs, 85 percent answered positively.

As the Society celebrated its fiftieth year, health journalist Jane Brody wrote a lengthy article in the *New York Times* describing progress against the disease that she attributed "to the support for research from the indefatigable Lawry." Brody concluded, "Judging from the accelerating pace of research, experts believe that long before another 50 years have passed, there will be effective ways to help nearly all who develop multiple sclerosis to avoid or recover from the crippling destruction of myelin that is the hallmark of the disease."

Shortly after that *Times* article appeared, Sylvia Lawry received an unexpected phone call from Richard Owen, the son of Carl Owen, the first president of the Society. Now a federal judge in New York, the younger Owen told her, "At our dinner table at home, my father would often talk about how wonderful you were. I want you to know that even back then, people like my father recognized just what an extraordinary person you are."

Sylvia was almost speechless. "Well," she finally said, "when your father died, I thought that was the end of the world. I didn't know how we could continue without him."

Judge Owen replied, "My father believed it was you who was indispensable to the MS Society."

Despite the successes of the National MS Society, the organization's leaders recognize that there is always room for improvement. As a result, the National Society announced in 1999 that it had commissioned a twenty-month-long study by the prestigious National Academy of Sciences / Institute of Medicine to conduct a strategic review of MS. An expert panel of scientists and physicians will analyze the present knowledge of the causes and treatment of the disease, and recommend strategies to be pursued.

39

As Joseph Hartzler watched the news and the horrifying scenes of the bombing of the Alfred P. Murrah Federal Building in Oklahoma City in April 1995, the veteran U.S. prosecutor felt he needed to do something. "I thought I could make a difference," he said.

He had recently returned from a visit to the White House, where he met with President Clinton and was honored as the 1995 MS Father of the Year. But after Attorney General Janet Reno appointed him to head the eight-person prosecutorial team that would eventually win the conviction of bombing suspect Timothy McVeigh, the forty-four-year-old Hartzler brought multiple sclerosis into even greater public awareness. As he arrived at the courtroom on a motorized scooter each morning, he was undisturbed by the crowds and always professional in his demeanor. As *Inside MS* observed, "Rarely has it been more clear that ability, not disability, counts."

Hartzler graduated summa cum laude from the American University Law School and had been the head of both the civil and criminal divisions of the U.S. Attorney's Office in Chicago.

He had been diagnosed with MS in the late 1980s but had never let it interfere with his life in significant ways. He coached his son's Little League team in Springfield, Illinois—a team called the Mighty Skunks, whose initials were a tongue-in-cheek play on his disease. Despite his professional accomplishments, Hartzler remained humble and soft-spoken—qualities that brought dignity to the judicial proceedings at the McVeigh bombing trial. As one fellow attorney said, "His integrity is beyond reproach."

In 1998 the Society named Hartzler, his wife Lisa, and their three sons MS Family of the Year. Lisa is an energetic fundraiser for the Society, and the entire family participates in the MS Walk.

Hartzler had spoken at the Society's National Leadership Conference in Dallas in 1997, where he said: "A lot of people have asked me how was it to have MS and handle all the stress of the Oklahoma trial. 'I don't really do stress,' I'd say. But what I really mean is . . . don't pity me. Pity is the last thing most of us need or want. Yes, I have MS and it affects me every day—every minute. But what's the point of dwelling on it? Life can be pretty good even with MS."

Hartzler continued, "MS is the Baskin-Robbins of chronic illness. It comes in such a wide variety of flavors. Another lawyer with MS told me he can feel his stress rising just thinking of the courtroom. Another lawyer with MS told me she goes into cognitive never-never land. But my symptoms are largely mobility-related. I don't have cognitive slowdown. So while I've been a poster boy for MS and I hope I've helped a lot of people understand more about the disease, I'm afraid I've also been the source of: 'Hey, he can do that, so get your butt off the couch and do it, too.' I could do what I did because I have a limited number of symptoms. I haven't found it easy, but I have learned to accept my disability. I have never learned to accept that there is no cure. I'm beginning to think I might not have to."

The enormous attention surrounding Hartzler during the McVeigh trial helped the nation and the world to better understand multiple sclerosis and the capabilities of people with the disease. In another major and ongoing story of the 1990s, the media portrayed a different side of MS—the despair of some people with the disease—as it recounted the controversial physician-assisted-suicide activities of Dr. Jack Kevorkian. The Michigan-based pathologist believed that people with chronic illnesses that cause enormous suffering have the right to choose to die with dignity. Several of his patients had MS, including a fifty-four-year-old woman who had been diagnosed a decade earlier. She could no longer engage in the activities of life that she had enjoyed—from hooking rugs to shopping at the mall. She couldn't afford a full-time nurse or an electric wheelchair, and she had become incontinent. At that point she chose death over life, and Kevorkian was there to assist her.

In response to the attention paid to Kevorkian's activities, *Inside MS* devoted part of its Summer 1996 issue to the subject. Pamela Cavallo, the Society's director of clinical programs, noted, "I've led many groups of people with MS in discussions about suicide. They almost always start with tremendous anger. People say, 'We struggle every day. They gave up!' Yet there are suicides every day by people who don't have MS. We need to put the issue in perspective."

Ms. Cavallo emphasized that most suicides are not MS-related, but she conceded that chronic illness is a major risk factor for the general population. "So, by definition, people with MS are at some risk."

The Kevorkian controversy also prompted the National Society to issue a position statement: "The foundation of our mission lies in our deep concern for people with MS and their families and our awareness of how difficult life with this disease can be. The National Multiple Sclerosis Society cares about people with MS who consider suicide. We respect our clients' right to self-determination. At the same time, the Society affirms life and offers programs and services which promote positive coping with chronic disease."

Living with MS can pose enormous challenges, including many that are still poorly understood even by physicians. In the foreword to a 1999 book, *Women Living with Multiple Sclerosis,* Robert M. Reed, M.D., wrote, "As a neurologist, I have been caring for people with multiple sclerosis for 25 years, but until reading this book I never fully understood the depth of suffering the patient with MS endures."

Nevertheless the spirit of people with MS is undeniable. Florida resident Courtney Watson met another person with MS—a woman named April from Arkansas—on the Internet, and the two of them began corresponding via e-mail each day. Though they had never met, they decided that the 1997 MS Walk would be the perfect place to do so. But two weeks before the event, Courtney's disease began to relapse. In tears, she called April to let her know that she might not be able to participate. April told her, "Yes you will. Even if I have to push you in a wheelchair, we will do this walk and finish it together!"

April was right. They both were able to walk. And they finished together.

Family members know very well just how challenging it can be living with MS. Marion Marx, a resident of Birmingham, Alabama, supported her sister's courageous battle against the disease, and Marion and Sylvia Lawry struck up a friendship through the mail. "I encouraged her to organize a Birmingham chapter," said Sylvia.

In one of Sylvia's notes to Ms. Marx, she mentioned how she was "reliving the trials of the early days as I raise money for the International Federation." Several months later a holiday card arrived from Marion, which included a check for $50,000 made out to the International Federation and targeted for scientific research. The donation was in memory of Marion's sister.

Even though MS can sometimes pose many obstacles to a normal life, persons with the disease are typically driven more by hope than by hopelessness. Marsha Moers, winner of the MS Achiever of 1996 Award, had such rapidly progressing MS that she was forced into a nursing home at the age of thirty-five. But eventually she was able to move home, with the help of a part-time aide. She began to work as an advocate for people with disabilities and volunteer at her local MS chapter.

When Marsha accepted her award at the International Leadership Conference in Atlanta, she said, "When I was in college, I pledged the very best sorority. We were the brightest and most ambitious young women at the school. There wasn't anything we couldn't do. But the kid who had all the promise just didn't exist after MS. It took me a long time to learn that the kid I used to be wasn't dead after all. Here I am, I have a family, friends, a community. I have accomplishments I'm proud of. And I can tell my sorority sisters, 'Look at me now!'"

Then Marsha added, "I can say to all my brothers and sisters who also struggle with MS: Yes, there is hope. Yes, we have a right to have great expectations for ourselves."

Those great expectations are an integral part of Zoe Koplowitz's life. She has made participating in the New York City

Marathon an annual ritual since 1988, and has turned it into "the journey of a lifetime." It has become a metaphor for her own triumph over disability. In 2000, walking with the help of crutches, she finished the grueling 26.2-mile course in 33 hours, the last person to complete the event! She is the *Guinness Book of World Records* titleist in this category.

MS, said Zoe, has taught her a lot—patience, humor, discipline, and humility. When she spoke at the Society's National Leadership Conference, she said, "Many of you run marathons every day, just by getting up and saying 'yes.' 'Yes' is one of the shortest words in the English language and one of the biggest. It is full of possibility and power and pleasure." In her book, *The Winning Spirit,* she describes herself as the human Post-it note you stick to your refrigerator to remind yourself, "You can do it!"

40

"WHAT MIND can conceive, man can achieve."
Sylvia Lawry came across that credo many years ago and chose it as her own. For decades she believed that multiple sclerosis would be conquered, though in the earliest days of the Society, most physicians considered it to be a disease without hope. Some people with MS were treated with herbs and bed rest. Others were told that they were mentally ill, and were even subjected to brain surgery to cure their illness.

But times have changed for the better for people with multiple sclerosis. In almost every community, people with MS can find a doctor with expertise in caring for the disease. A few drugs can influence the underlying course of MS and significantly improve the lives of patients. Many services are now available that back in the forties and fifties were unthinkable. Public attitudes toward disabilities have improved, and thanks to laws like the Americans with Disabilities Act, individuals with MS now have more protection at the workplace and greater accessibility to public buildings. Most persons with MS can now realistically expect to have a normal life expectancy. Fewer than one in four will ever become totally disabled and use a wheel-chair. And there are reasons for even greater optimism about the future. Still, Mike Dugan has said, "We must speed up pos-itive change and stop unfavorable change. I'm not content with the state of the MS world today, and neither are you."

John McGillicuddy, chairman emeritus of the National So-ciety, once said, "I would love to get to the point where we have a major controversy in the Society. And that controversy would be, 'Now that we've found a cure for MS, do we disband or go on to tackle something else?' That's my dream."

Some people still look upon the Salk polio vaccine as the type of breakthrough that MS needs. They use the word "cure" when they talk about the ultimate goal. But the debate goes on over whether a "cure" is realistic for those who already have the disease. "Cure implies reversal," said Dugan. "No one who was paralyzed with polio ever got up from his or her wheelchair and walked because of the Salk vaccine. When it comes to MS, I believe something significant will happen in the next five years. There are many areas where investments are being made, and there is great potential for making significant progress against the disease. I dream that we will first develop something that stabilizes MS." Halting the progression of the disease would satisfy many people with MS, along with the prospect of improvement through rehabilitation.

Dr. W. Ian McDonald of the Multiple Sclerosis Interna-tional Federation pointed out that while there are still impor-tant questions to be answered in every major area related to MS, research is moving ahead at a faster pace than ever before. "There were important conceptual advances in the nineties, whereas not much had really changed in the previous thirty years."

While the degeneration of nerve cells (in addition to the

damage to myelin) has been known to exist in MS for more than a century, only in the 1990s did researchers generally agree that this process is probably an important factor in producing the disability that occurs with the disease. "If we understand exactly how the neurons are damaged so that they degenerate, there would be the possibility of developing strategies for preventing degeneration," said Dr. McDonald. "The whole field of neuroprotection is a very exciting one, with rapid progress being made." According to Dr. McDonald, there is good evidence that long-term disability is influenced by the frequency and severity of inflammatory attacks. "So if we could stop the inflammation from occurring, we could stop new disability from developing."

In 1996, Mike Dugan predicted, "Over the next ten years, I firmly believe we will be able to regulate the course of MS for most people. People with MS will be recognized for their abilities and contributions and their presence will be routine in the workplace. . . . I also expect we will have multiple therapeutic interventions against the effects of MS. I have a vision of a world that is finally free of this disease. Hard work and good decisions will get us there."

As of 2000, the National MS Society had invested more than $310 million into MS research. In addition, it had promoted growth in National Institutes of Health investments in MS to the $120 million mark per year. Stephen Reingold, vice president of research programs for the National Society, emphasizes that science doesn't work in a predictable fashion. But he believes that in the next five to ten years, "We'll understand the genetics of MS, and we'll be able to have a significant impact on the progression of disability. We'll see efforts to take what we've learned and move it to the clinical setting, perhaps trying to actually encourage the recovery function."

Dr. McDonald believes that research may lead to a way to restore function in some persons with MS. "This might be possible someday, most likely in people with partial damage, where some nerve fibers concerned with a particular function still survive," he said. "We might be able to promote activity of the surviving cells. Suppose you've got a very weak foot, which is not uncommon; for regeneration to occur, we must find a way to stimulate nerve regrowth in the right place, which is in the muscles of the foot. That will be a challenge, but it is a feasible proposition. Fortunately, particularly in the earlier stages of MS, there is only partial damage at that point, so some kind of restoration function may be possible."

Dr. Stanley van den Noort, chief medical officer of the National MS Society, concurs that the potential for regrowing nerve cells and regrowing myelin exist. "It's likely that we will develop growth factors that can do this," he said. "Much more research needs to be done, but we're beginning to make headway. It's a very exciting area of study."

The availability of the "A-B-C" drugs—Avonex, Betaseron, and Copaxone—has been a major breakthrough, added Dr. van den Noort. "The fact that we've gotten three partial answers to MS in the last ten years astounds me. I'm so thrilled that we have them. And there will be new drugs—a lot of them—in the future. Yes, we need better drugs, but they're coming along."

One of the newest medications added to the MS arsenal is Novantrone (or mitoxantrone), which the FDA approved in October 2000 for "reducing neurologic disability and/or the frequency of clinical relapses" in individuals with secondary-progressive, progressive-relapsing, or worsening relapsing-remitting MS. It is the first drug approved in the United States for treating the secondary-progressive form of the disease, and is administered every three months via an infusion into the vein.

The assault on MS has become more aggressive in other ways. A $1 million gift from the family of Richard Slifka, national board chairman, is being used to fund the first comprehensive study that will follow a representative sample of two thousand persons with MS over a long period of time. The Sonya Slifka Longitudinal Multiple Sclerosis Study was named for Richard's mother, who had MS. It will collect data on clinical characteristics, prognostic factors, treatment approaches, quality of life, family concerns, and other issues.

The Mount Sinai School of Medicine and the Mount Sinai Hospital in New York are establishing the Corrine (Corky) Goldsmith Dickinson Center for Multiple Sclerosis, thanks to a $5 million gift from George J. Gillespie and Clifford Goldsmith, both former chairmen of the National MS Society. The center, named for Goldsmith's daughter (who died of MS in 1999), will provide a site for comprehensive patient care and research related to MS. Gillespie and Goldsmith expressed their resolve that "Corky's Center" will "make a significant contribution to the lives of those stricken with this cruel disease both in treatment and finally a cure." The new facility is expected to recruit leaders in MS research worldwide to provide the scientific innovation that can ultimately conquer the disease.

Sylvia Lawry often looked back upon her own long commitment to the cause and wished that all the answers to MS were at hand. Some people in the movement had thrown up their hands in frustration and drifted away. "But," said Sylvia, "others realize that much more funding and public awareness have been channeled into solving the cancer problem, for instance, and the solution to cancer still hasn't come. So there's no need for us to be defensive." As Dr. Harry Weaver once put it, "MS is a far more complex problem than I, a scientist, had ever realized."

When the ultimate breakthroughs are finally made, history will record the crucial role of the National MS Society and the International Federation in those achievements. "The goal that I've always had has not yet been accomplished," said Sylvia. "Sometimes, I think we could have done better if more funds had been available; we could have been more aggressive and perhaps more targeted in our approach. But the positives and the progress we've made far outweigh the negatives. The Society has helped so many people with MS and their families, and that has given me great consolation along the way."

Many people have recognized Sylvia's enormous contribution to the movement. Clarence Francis, the head of General Foods, was one of them. When Sylvia first met public relations guru Edward Bernays in the early days of the Society, he told her, "If you can get Clarence Francis to chair a fundraising dinner for the Society, no business leader in the U.S. would turn you down." Francis had been selected by the Rockefeller family to lead the campaign to build Lincoln Center in New York, and his influence in the corporate world was legendary.

Francis eventually became chairman of the National MS Society's National Advisory Council. He once told Sylvia, "You should keep notes about everything you're doing so you can write a book someday. The public should know that Horatio Alger is still alive." Her response: "I'm too busy making things happen to write about them!"

Not surprisingly, Sylvia always felt that she had something much more important to do than write a book—namely, to continue her irrevocable dedication to conquering multiple sclerosis. Along the way she made many personal sacrifices to lead the campaign against MS. She gave up her dreams of pursuing a legal career. She sometimes said that the long hours she spent in the national office too often stole her away from spending time with her children. She would have wanted to become a better tennis player and golfer, enjoy her home more, and travel to places she hadn't yet explored just for the joy of it, not because there were people in other parts of the country or the world with whom she had to meet to propel the movement forward.

In addition to many thousands of thank-yous that Sylvia received over the years, she was the recipient of more formal acknowledgments as well. For twenty-three years she served on the board of directors of the National Health Council, the organization composed of all the major voluntary health agencies, as well as government and business groups in the health field. The NHC presented Sylvia with an award for distinguished public service—the first award of its kind in the council's ninety-year history, and one she shared with a colleague on the NHC board. Because she had developed a model voluntary health agency, she was asked by the NHC to serve as a volunteer consultant to troubled member agencies. She also was often asked for guidance by other emerging organizations and from time to time was even invited to sit on their boards. She would politely decline such invitations, explaining, "No thanks, my heart belongs to beating multiple sclerosis."

In 1998 a formal portrait of Sylvia, painted by Pamela Bowman, was unveiled and now hangs in the lobby of the Society's home office in New York. In her remarks at the unveiling, Sylvia stressed that her dream had remained steadfast—to "live to see the day when the devastating effects of MS are conquered." If this were not realized in her lifetime, she added, she would be comforted by the fact that her portrait would serve to tap the conscience of those who survived her.

When Sylvia was once asked when she planned to retire, she responded, "I'll retire when MS retires."

"There wouldn't have been a National MS Society without her," said Mike Dugan. Judy Rahmani, the 1994 MS Mother of the Year, observed, "Sylvia Lawry may not yet have found the cure for MS, but she has assisted everyone touched by this devastating disease to deal and heal with it. She is a woman who has never sought personal recognition but who deserves it more than anyone I've ever met."

Alexis de Tocqueville, the nineteenth-century French statesman, was taken with America's character—the sense of humanity and the belief that individuals could effect change. These characteristics are chiefly responsible for volunteer movements in the United States and for the achievements of organizations like the National MS Society. They were also the driving force behind Sylvia Lawry, the Society's most committed volunteer, whose resolve helped stimulate the research that will ultimately bring MS to its knees. As Dr. Reingold said, "The research approach to MS, more than ever before, is broad-based and multidisciplinary, involving thousands of scientists and physicians around the world. This effort is going to make the difference."

Many years ago there was a minor rebellion among MS families in Columbus, Ohio, who talked of creating another national society dedicated to multiple sclerosis. Sylvia flew there in hopes of convincing them to join with the National MS Society instead. She met with the families and with some of the city's leading dignitaries, including Charles Lazarus of the Federated Department Stores, whose brother-in-law had multiple sclerosis. He had sponsored the local group, unaware of the existence of the National MS Society. Sylvia used her persuasiveness and worked her magic, and ended up quieting the rebellious spirit before it had really gotten very far. Today the National Society still serves people with MS from the office in Columbus.

As one of Lazarus's aides, Trent Sickles, drove Sylvia to the airport to return to New York, he could see the exhaustion in her face. When she was about to board the plane, Sickles remarked to her in Swedish, "Nicht legg lo." Sylvia didn't understand, but later she learned that it meant "Never give up."

Sylvia had those words engraved on a plaque and framed, and they held a prominent place on the wall in front of her desk.

"Never give up!" Sylvia said as she pointed to the plaque. "I look at it frequently. It's a constant reminder that when we have problems, there has got to be a solution. That's how I feel about the fight against MS. I'll never give up."

Afterword

"MULTIPLE SCLEROSIS. *Will anyone recovered from it please communicate with patient . . .*"—words that changed the world for people with MS and their families.

THE HISTORY of the crusade against multiple sclerosis is truly the story of Sylvia Lawry and the millions of people she energized and inspired to battle this complex, devastating disease. In the beginning it was a personal effort focused on her brother, but gradually, inexorably, it grew into a lifelong quest on behalf of a much wider audience; it became a calling, a much larger mission—to rid the world of MS.

In the fifty-six years since she placed her singular and unconventional inquiry in the *New York Times*, the world has witnessed extraordinary changes politically, economically, technologically, and socially, but for people with MS and their families these changes have not transformed their lives proportionately.

Some important things have changed: early diagnosis; a wide array of effective symptomatic treatments; individual and group social support; extensive and constantly updated lay and professional publications; and the mobilization of thousands of researchers in academic and pharmaceutical settings pursuing the causes and treatment of MS. All of these accomplishments are due to Sylvia Lawry's vision, dedication, and determination.

While we celebrate these achievements, there remain obstacles and challenges yet to be overcome. Although the first, partially effective therapeutic interventions became available in the mid-1990s, an understanding of exactly what precipitates MS continues to be indescribable; drugs that are fully effective for a broad cross section of those diagnosed with the disease lie in the future; a preventive regimen, or perhaps a vaccine, is yet to be demonstrated; and the ultimate dream—restoration of function—remains elusive.

After a lifetime of leading the struggle against multiple sclerosis, Sylvia Lawry succumbed to the even more intractable effects of age and infirmity. She joined the immortals on February 24, 2001.

Sylvia participated fully in the development of this book and was eager for its impending publication, not as a personal tribute but as a vehicle for broadening the public exposure of a little-known, difficult human condition and for attracting wider support to help accelerate the work necessary to overcome MS. Her mission continues.

Those who are fortunate enough to have known Sylvia Lawry salute her vision, her strength, her persistence, her will, and her selflessness. She was, indeed, a woman of courage.

MIKE DUGAN
friend and follower;
General, United States Air Force, Retired;
President and Chief Executive Officer,
National Multiple Sclerosis Society

Appendices

Appendix A
National Multiple Sclerosis Society
National Offices and Chapters (U.S.A.)

Mr. Richard B. Slifka, National Chairman
General Mike Dugan, USAF, Ret., President and CEO

National Offices

**National Multiple Sclerosis
  Society**
New York Center
733 Third Avenue
New York, NY 10017-3288
Tel: 212-986-3240

**National Multiple Sclerosis
  Society**
Public Policy Center
1100 New York Avenue, NW,
  Suite 1015
Washington, DC 20005
Tel: 202-408-1500

**National Multiple Sclerosis
  Society**
Training & Resource Center
700 Broadway, Suite 810
Denver, CO 80203
Tel: 303-813-1052

Chapter Offices

Alabama Chapter
3530 Independence Drive, Suite 3534
Birmingham, AL 35209
Tel: 205-879-8881
Mr. Anthony J. Tanner, Chair
Ms. Tracy Smith, Chapter President

Desert Southwest Chapter
315 South 48th Street, #101
Tempe, AZ 85281
Tel: 480-968-2488
Mr. James H. Bolin, Chair
Mr. Allen Gjersvig, Chapter President

Channel Islands Chapter
14 West Valerio Street
Santa Barbara, CA 93101
Tel: 805-682-8783
Mr. James Carder, Chair
Ms. Joan Young, Chapter President

Mountain Valley California Chapter
2277 Watt Avenue, Suite 300
Sacramento, CA 95825
Tel: 916-486-8981
Mr. Kenneth A. Lentsch, Chair
Ms. Barbara Dupree, Chapter President

Northern California Chapter
150 Grand Avenue
Oakland, CA 94612
Tel: 510-268-0572
Ms. Kathleen McEligot, Chair
Ms. Julie Thomas, Chapter President

Orange County Chapter
17500 Redhill Avenue, Suite 240
Irvine, CA 92614
Tel: 949-752-1680
Mr. Bill Bisch, Chair
Ms. Jamie MacDonald, Chapter President

Southern California Chapter
2440 South Sepulveda Boulevard, Suite 115
Los Angeles, CA 90064
Tel: 310-479-4456
Mr. Robert E. Harper, Chair
Mr. Leon LeBuffe, Chapter President

San Diego Area Chapter
8840 Complex Drive, Suite 130
San Diego, CA 92123
Tel: 858-974-8640
Ms. Hope Anderson, Chair
Mr. Allan Shaw, Chapter President

Silicon Valley Chapter
2589 Scott Boulevard
Santa Clara, CA 95050
Tel: 408-988-7557
Dr. Patricia Hanley-Peterson,
  Chair
Ms. Carla Hines, Chapter
  President

Colorado Chapter
700 Broadway, Suite 808
Denver, CO 80203
Tel: 303-831-0700
Ms. Janet Savage, Chair
Ms. Dianne Williams, Chapter
  President

Greater Connecticut Chapter
705 North Mountain Road,
  Suite G102
Newington, CT 06111
Tel: 860-953-0601
Mr. Jack Weber, Chair
Ms. Lisa Gerrol, Chapter
  President

Western Connecticut Chapter
One Selleck Street, Suite 500
Norwalk, CT 06855
Tel: 203-838-1033
Mr. Peter Porrino, Chair
Ms. M. Elizabeth Fairbanks,
  Chapter President

National Capital Chapter
2021 K Street, NW, Suite 715
Washington, DC 20006
Tel: 202-296-5363
Mr. Lee Stillwell, Chair
Ms. Jeanne Oates Angulo,
  Chapter President

Delaware Chapter
Two Mill Road, Suite 106
Wilmington, DE 19806
Tel: 302-655-5610
Mr. Henry Morneau, Chair
Ms. Kate Cowperthwait, Chapter
  President

Mid-Florida Chapter
3659 Maguire Boulevard,
  Suite 110
Orlando, FL 32803
Tel: 407-896-3873
Ms. Cathy Kerns, Chair
Ms. Tami Caesar, Chapter
  President

North Florida Chapter
9550 Regency Square
  Boulevard, Suite 104
Jacksonville, FL 32225
Tel: 904-725-6800
Mr. J. Daniel Baker, Chair
Ms. Jennifer Lee, Chapter
  President

South Florida Chapter
5450 N.W. 33rd Avenue,
  Suite 110
Fort Lauderdale, FL 33309
Tel: 954-731-4224
Mr. Joey Epstein, Chair
Ms. Karen Dresbach, Chapter
  President

Georgia Chapter
12 Perimeter Center East,
 Suite 1200
Atlanta, GA 30346
Tel: 770-393-8833
Mr. Chelton D. Tanger, Chair
Ms. Mary Creighton, Chapter
 President

Iowa Chapter
1300 50th Street, Suite 106
West Des Moines, IA 50266-
 5499
Tel: 515-270-6337
Mr. Richard Bice, Chair
Mr. Brett Ridge, Chapter
 President

Greater Illinois Chapter
910 West Van Buren Street, 4th
 Floor
Chicago, IL 60607
Tel: 312-421-4500
Ms. Nanciann Huening, Chair
Mr. Steven Pratapas, Chapter
 President

Indiana State Chapter
7301 Georgetown Road,
 Suite 112
Indianapolis, IN 46268
Tel: 317-870-2500
Ms. Vicki Yamasaki, Chair
Ms. Theresa Brun, Chapter
 President

Mid-America Chapter
5442 Martway
Shawnee Mission, KS 66205
Tel: 913-432-3926
Ms. Anne Canfield, Chair
Ms. Kay Julian Coe, Chapter
 President

**Kentucky/Southeast Indiana
 Chapter**
1169 Eastern Parkway,
 Suite 2266
Louisville, KY 40217
Tel: 502-451-0014
Ms. Shirley Powers, Chair
Ms. Dawn Lee, Chapter
 President

Louisiana Chapter
3616 South I-10 Service Road,
 Suite 101
Metairie, LA 70001
Tel: 504-832-4013
Mr. Robert E. Howson, Chair
Ms. Karen McGuire, Chapter
 President

Central New England Chapter
101A First Avenue, Suite 6
Waltham, MA 02451
Tel: 781-890-4990
Mr. William Keough, Chair
Ms. Arlyn White, Chapter
 President

Maryland Chapter
Hunt Valley Business Center
10946 Beaver Dam Road,
  Suite E
Cockeysville, MD 21030
Tel: 410-527-1770
Mr. Stephen Zentz, Chair
Mr. Rick Smith, Chapter
  President

Maine Chapter
P.O. Box 8730
Portland, ME 04104
Tel: 207-761-5815
Mr. William Dunn, Chair
Ms. Susan Greenwood, Chapter
  President

Michigan Chapter
21311 Civic Center Drive
Southfield, MI 48076
Tel: 248-350-0020
Dr. Stanton Elias, Chair
Ms. Patricia McDonald, Chapter
  President

Minnesota Chapter
200 12th Avenue South
Minneapolis, MN 55415
Tel: 612-335-7900
Mr. Richard A. Knutson, Chair
Ms. Maureen Reeder, Chapter
  President

Gateway Area Chapter
1867 Lackland Hill Parkway
St. Louis, MO 63146
Tel: 314-781-9020
Ms. Jacquelyn L. Dezort, Chair
Ms. Patricia Knoerle-Jordan,
  Chapter President

Central North Carolina
  Chapter
2211 West Meadowview Road,
  Suite 30
Greensboro, NC 27407
Tel: 336-299-4136
Mr. Scott Greer, Chair
Ms. Elizabeth Ruffin-Green,
  Chapter President

Eastern North Carolina
  Chapter
3101 Industrial Drive, Suite 210
Raleigh, NC 27609
Tel: 919-834-0678
Mr. Milo Brunick, Chair
Ms. Robin Boettcher, Chapter
  President

Mid-Atlantic Chapter
9844 C Southern Pines Blvd.
Charlotte, NC 28273
Tel: 704-525-2955
Mr. Mike Daisley, Chair
Ms. Anne Marie McDermott,
  Chapter President

Nebraska Chapter
Community Health Plaza
7101 Newport Avenue,
  Suite 203
Omaha, NE 68152
Tel: 402-572-3190
Mr. David Gilinsky, Chair
Ms. Patricia Gorham, Chapter
  President

Greater North Jersey Chapter
1 Kalisa Way, Suite 205
Paramus, NJ 07652
Tel: 201-967-5599
Mr. Thomas M. Rosen, Chair
Ms. Nancy P. Lorenzi, Chapter
President

Mid-Jersey Chapter
246 Monmouth Road
Oakhurst, NJ 07755
Tel: 732-660-1005
Mr. Terry C. Moncrief, Chair
Mr. Michael Elkow, Chapter
President

Great Basin Sierra Chapter
1201 Terminal Way, Suite 215
Reno, NV 89502
Tel: 775-329-7180
Ms. Jan Hermsen, Chair
Ms. Lynne Sunderman, Chapter
President

Long Island Chapter
200 Parkway Drive South, #101
Hauppauge, NY 11788
Tel: 631-864-8337
Mr. Eugene DeMark, Chair
Ms. Johanna Biederman,
Chapter President

**Northeastern New York
Chapter**
9 Columbia Circle
Albany, NY 12203
Tel: 518-464-0630
Ms. Ellie Kittle-Ingalsbe, Chair
Ms. Barbara Roland-Milano,
Chapter President

New York City Chapter
30 West 26th Street, 9th Floor
New York, NY 10010
Tel: 212-463-7787
Mr. Frank Brown, Chair
Ms. Carol Kurzig, Chapter
President

Southern New York Chapter
2 Gannett Drive, Suite LC
White Plains, NY 10604
Tel: 914-694-1655
Ms. Mary Foster, Chair
Mr. Ken Mongold, Chapter
President

Upstate New York Chapter
1650 South Avenue, Suite 100
Rochester, NY 14620
Tel: 716-271-0801
Mr. Richard Kazel, Chair
Mr. James Ahearn, Chapter
President

**West New York/Northwest
Pennsylvania Chapter**
4245 Union Road, Suite 108
Buffalo, NY 14225
Tel: 716-634-2261
Mr. Ronald Tanski, Chair
Mr. Arthur Cardella, Chapter
President

Mid-Ohio Chapter
970 Crupper Avenue
Columbus, OH 43229
Tel: 614-880-2290

Northeast Ohio Chapter
The Hanna Building
1422 Euclid Avenue, Suite 333
Cleveland, OH 44115
Tel: 216-696-8220
Mr. John Simonetti, Chair
Ms. Janet Kramer, Chapter
President

Northwest Ohio Chapter
401 Tomahawk Drive
Maumee, OH 43537
Tel: 419-897-9533
Mr. J. R. Toland, Chair
Ms. Jeanette Hrovatich, Chapter
President

Southwest Ohio/North
Kentucky Chapter
4460 Lake Forest Drive,
Suite 236
Cincinnati, OH 45242
Tel: 513-769-4400
Ms. Dianne Bohmer, Chair
Ms. Tena Bunnell, Chapter
President

Western Ohio Chapter
The Woolpert Building
409 East Monument, Suite 101
Dayton, OH 45402
Tel: 937-461-5232
Ms. Judy LaMusga, Chair

Oklahoma Chapter
4606 East 67th Street, Suite 103
Tulsa, OK 74136
Tel: 918-488-0882
Mr. Kevin O'Sullivan, Chair
Ms. Paula Cortner, Chapter
President

Oregon Chapter
1650 N.W. Naito Avenue,
Suite 190
Portland, OR 97209
Tel: 503-223-9511
Ms. Laura Black, Chair
Ms. Carol Vogel, Chapter
President

Allegheny District Chapter
1040 Fifth Avenue, 2nd Floor
Pittsburgh, PA 15219
Tel: 412-261-6347
Mr. Samuel S. Zacharias, Chair
Ms. Colleen McGuire, Chapter
President

Central Pennsylvania Chapter
2209 Forest Hills Drive, #18
Harrisburg, PA 17112
Tel: 717-652-2108
Mr. Walter Froh, Chair
Ms. Margie Adelmann, Chapter
President

Greater Delaware Valley
Chapter
1 Reed Street
Philadelphia, PA 19147
Tel: 215-271-2400
Mr. Kent C. Griswold, Chair
Ms. Judith Cohen, Chapter
President

Rhode Island Chapter
205 Hallene Road, Suite 209
Warwick, RI 02886
Tel: 401-738-8383
Mr. Eric Emerson, Chair
Ms. Kathy Mechnig, Chapter
President

Dakota Chapter
1000 East 41st Street
Sioux Falls, SD 57105
Tel: 605-336-7017
Ms. Jan Feterl, Chair
Ms. Kathie Brown, Chapter
  President

Mid-South Chapter
6685 Quince Road, Suite 124
Memphis, TN 38119
Tel: 901-755-4900
Mr. Edwin Barnett, Chair
Ms. Helen Feinstein, Chapter
  President

Middle Tennessee Chapter
4219 Hillsboro Road, Suite 306
Memphis, TN 37215
Tel: 615-269-9055
Mr. Kevin Poff, Chair
Mr. Jim Ward, Chapter President

**Southeast Tennessee/North
  Georgia Chapter**
5720 Uptain Road, Suite 4800
Chattanooga, TN 37411
Tel: 423-954-9700
Mr. Sean McMurray, Chair
Mr. Glenn Czarnecki, Chapter
  President

Lone Star Chapter
8111 North Stadium Drive,
  Suite 100
Houston, TX 77054
Tel: 713-526-8967
Dr. Raymond A. Martin, Chair
Ms. Pat Bertotti, Chapter
  President

North Central Texas Chapter
4086 Sandshell Drive
Fort Worth, TX 76137
Tel: 817-306-7003
Mr. Cary Dorman, Chair
Ms. Evelyn Taylor, Chapter
  President

Panhandle Chapter
6222 Canyon Drive
Amarillo, TX 79109
Tel: 806-468-7500
Mr. William P. Harris, Chair
Ms. Jeri Farris, Chapter
  President

Utah State Chapter
2995 S.W. Temple, Suite C
Salt Lake City, UT 84115
Tel: 801-493-0113
Mr. Pete Taylor, Chair
Ms. Tami Featherstone, Chapter
  President

Blue Ridge Chapter
1 Morton Drive, Suite 106
Charlottesville, VA 22903
Tel: 804-971-0810
Mr. Donald Sandridge, Chair
Ms. Faith Painter, Chapter
  President

Central Virginia Chapter
1301 North Hamilton Street,
  Suite 108
Richmond, VA 23230
Tel: 804-353-5008
Ms. Beverly Snukals, Chair
Ms. Connie McKenzie Hedrick,
  Chapter President

Hampton Roads Chapter
405 South Parliament Drive,
  Suite 105
Virginia Beach, VA 23462
Tel: 757-490-9627
Mr. D. R. Carpenter, Chair
Ms. Sharon Grossman, Chapter
  President

Greater Washington Chapter
192 Nickerson Street, Suite 100
Seattle, WA 98109
Tel: 206-284-4236
Mr. Jim O'Donnell, Chair
Ms. Patricia Shepherd-Barnes,
  Chapter President

Inland Northwest Chapter
818 East Sharp
Spokane, WA 99202
Tel: 509-482-2022
Ms. Sharon Van Auch, Chair
Mr. Robert Hansen, Chapter
  President

Wisconsin Chapter
W223 N608 Saratoga Drive,
  Suite 110
Waukesha, WI 53186
Tel: 262-547-8999
Mr. Morry L. Birnbaum, Chair
Ms. Colleen Kalt, Chapter
  President

Appendix B
Multiple Sclerosis International Federation

Esclerosis Multiple Argentina
  Asociacion
Uriarte 1465/69
1414 Buenos Aires
ARGENTINA
Tel: (54) 11 4 831 6617
Nadine Vila Moret, Chief
  Executive

National MS Society of
  Australia
34 Jackson Lane
Toorak
Victoria 3142
AUSTRALIA
Tel: (613) 9828 7222
Lindsay McMillan, Executive
  Director

Osterreichische MS
  Gesellschaft
Neurolog. Univ. Klinik
A-1090 Wien
Wahringer Guertel 18–20
AUSTRIA
Tel: (43) 1 40400 3121
Ursula Hensel, Chief Executive

Ligue Nationale Belge
de la Sclerose en Plaques
Avenue Eugene Plasky,
  173/bte 11
B-1030 Bruxelles
BELGIUM
Tel: (32) 2 736 1638
Christiane Tihon, (Acting) Chief
  Executive

Assoc. Brasileira de EM
Rua Demostenes 283
04614-011 Sao Paulo, SP
BRAZIL
Tel: (55) 11 533 0582
Suely Berner, Chief Executive

MS Society of Canada
Suite 1000, 250 Bloor Street
  East
Toronto, Ontario M4W 3P9
CANADA
Tel: (1) 416 922 6065
Alistair M. Fraser, National
  President & Chief Executive

Cyprus MS Association
PO Box 6749
Nicosia 1647
CYPRUS
Tel: (357) 2 525 053
Celia Petridou, Secretary
  General

Unie Roska v CR Czech MS
  Society
PO Box 38
120 00 Praha 2
CZECH REPUBLIC
Tel: (420) 2 472 8619
Dr. Petr Lensky, Adviser

Scleroseforeningen
Mosedalvej 15
DK-2500 Valby
Copenhagen
DENMARK
Tel: (45) 364 63646
Peter Kauffeldt, Managing
  Director

The Finnish MS Society
Seppalantie 90, PL 15
FIN-21251 Masku
FINLAND
Tel: (358) 2 439 2111
Liisa Leiva, Executive Director

Ligue Francaise Contre la
  Sclérose en Plaq.
40, rue Duranton
75015 Paris
FRANCE
Tel: (33) 1 53 98 98 80
Vacancy, Chief Executive Officer

Deutsche Multiple Sklerose
  Gesellschaft
Vahrenwalder str. 205–207
30165 Hannover
GERMANY
Tel: (49) 511 96 8340
Dorothea Pitschnau, M.A.,
  Secretary General

MS Society of Great Britain &
  Northern Ireland
372 Edgware Road
London
NW2 6ND
GREAT BRITAIN
Tel: (44) 020 8438 0700
Peter Cardy, Chief Executive

Greek MS Society
KAANA
Vouliagmenis Avenue
Hellinikon 167 77
Athens
GREECE
Tel: (301) 964 4166/7
Hara Papadopoulou, Chief
  Executive

MS Society of Hungary
c/o Central Hospital of County
Fejer
Department of Neurology
H-8001 Szekesfehervar
Seregelyesi ut. 3
HUNGARY
Tel: (36) 22 316001
Dr. Andras Guseo,
President/Chief Executive

MS Felag Islands
Slettuvegur 5
103 Reykjavik
ICELAND
Tel: (354) 568 8620
Vilborg Traustadottir, Chief
Executive

MS Society of India (MSSI)
c/o Mrs. Sheela M. Chitnis
2nd Samata Sadan
S. H. Paralkar Road
Shivaji Park
Dadar—400 028
INDIA
Tel: (91) 444 2067
Mrs. Sheela M. Chitnis, Hon.
Secretary & National
Coordinator

MS Society of Ireland
Royal Hospital Donnybrook
Bloomfield Avenue
Morehampton Road, Dublin 4
IRELAND
Tel: (353) 1 269 4599
Michael Dineen, Chief Executive

Israel MS Society
75 Yehuda Halevi Street
Tel Aviv 65796
ISRAEL
Tel: (972) 3 560 9222
Janine Vosburgh, Executive
Director

Assoc. Italiana Sclerosi Multipla
Vico Chiuso Paggi 3
16128 Genova
ITALY
Tel: (39) 010 27131
Mario Alberto Battaglia, CEO

Japan MS Society
4-1-2 Kotobuki
Taitoku, Tokyo
JAPAN
Tel: (81) 3 3847 3504
Mr. Yasushi Nishimura,
Secretary General

Latvijas Multiplas Sklerozes
Asociacijas (LMSA)
1-104 Slokas Street
Riga
LV-1048
LATVIA
Tel: (371) 245 7605
Dr. Andrejs Millers, Chief
Executive

Ligue Luxembourgeoise
de la Sclérose en Plaques
boite postale 1444
L-1014 Luxembourg
LUXEMBOURG
Tel: (352) 400 844
Vacancy, Chief Executive

Multiple Sclerosis Society of
  Malta
PO Box 209
C.M.R.
Valletta
MALTA
(Associate Member)
Tel: (356) 418 066
Godfrey Leone Ganado, Vice
  President

Asociacion Mex contra
  Esclerosis
Multiple a.c.
Calzada de Tlalpan 4515
Tlalpan—Toriello Guerra
14050 Mexico D.F.
MEXICO
Tel: (52 5) 665 2022/0254
Ian Thomas, CEO/General
  Director

Multiple Sclerose Vereniging
  Nederland
Postbus 30470
2500 GL Den Haag
THE NETHERLANDS
Tel: (31) 70 374 77 77
Vacancy, Chief Executive

MS Society of New Zealand
  (Inc.)
PO Box 2627, Wellington
NEW ZEALAND
Tel: (64) 4 499 4677
Trudi Jordan, Executive
  Director

Multiple Sklerose Forbundet I
  Norge
Sorkedalsveien 3
0369 Oslo
NORWAY
Tel: (47) 22 604 960
Arnt Holte, Chief Executive

MS Society of Poland
(Polskie Towarzvstwo
  Stwardnienia Rozsianego)
c/o Marriott Hotel
Al Jerozolimski 65/79
00-697 Warsaw
POLAND
Tel: (48) 22 630 7220
Maria Kassur, Secretary General

Sociedade Portuguesa de
  Esclerose Multipla
Rua Tomas Alcaide 63C
1900 Lisboa
PORTUGAL
Tel: (351) 21 837 6610
Jorge da Silva, Secretary General

Slovensky zvaz Sclerosis
  Multiplex (SZSM)
Vancurova 1
917 00 Trnava
SLOVAKIA
(Associate Member)
Tel: (421) 21 805 5513 009
Milan Surgoš, President

Zdruzenje MS Slovenije
Maroltova ul. 14
1113 Ljubljana
SLOVENIA
Tel: (386) 568 7299
Mateja De Reya, Secretary
  General

South African National MS
  Society
PO Box 91077, Auckland Park
  2006
Johannesburg
SOUTH AFRICA
Tel: (27) 21 794 3322
Isobel Henderson, Chief
  Executive

Asociacion Espanola de EM
  (AEDEM)
Modesto Lafuente
8 1° Centro Derecha
28010—Madrid
SPAIN
Tel: (34) 91 448 1261
Pedro de la Prida, Secretary
  General

NHR (Neurologiskt
  Handikappades Riksforbund)
PO Box 3284
S-103 65 Stockholm
SWEDEN
Tel: (46) 8 677 70 10
Stefan Kall, Chief Executive

Schweizerische MS Gesellschaft
Brinerstrassel
CH-8036 Zurich
SWITZERLAND
Tel: (41) 1 461 4600
Dr. Hans-Peter Fricker, Chief
  Executive Officer

Türkiye Multipl Skleroz
  Dernegi
Büyükdere Caddesi Hukukcular
  Sitesi
No. 24 Kat 2 Daire 21 80290
Mecidizeköy—Istanbul
TURKEY
Tel: (90) 212 275 22 96
Aysegul Unlusoy, Chief
  Executive

National MS Society
733 Third Avenue
New York, NY 10017
UNITED STATES
Tel: (1) (212) 986 3240
Mike Dugan, President, CEO

MS Society of Zimbabwe
PO Box BE 1234
Belvedere, Harare
ZIMBABWE
Tel: (263) 4 740 472
Michael Robinson, President

Index